# The Truth About Scars and Roadblocks to Healing

*What Every Patient, Doctor, and Surgeon Needs to Know*

## Shannon Eggleston
#1 Best Selling Author

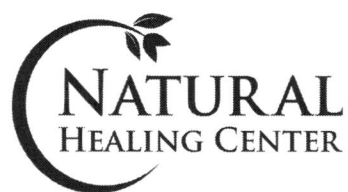

www.NaturalHealingCenter.US

---

**Fill out the systems survey and receive your free consultation!**

https://naturalhealingcenter.us/survey

*The Truth About Scars: What Every Patient, Surgeon, and Doctor Needs to Know.* Copyright © 2018 Shannon Eggleston

ISBN-13: 978-1718911239

All rights reserved. No part of this book may be used or reproduced in any manner whatsoever; nor may it be stored in a retrieval system, transmitted, or otherwise copied for public or private use - other than for "fair use" as brief quotations embodied in articles and reviews in their entirety - without written permission. For information, send an email to info@naturalhealingcenter.us

# TABLE OF CONTENTS

Introduction: Welcome to *The Truth About Scars and Roadblocks to Healing!* .................................... 1

Endorsements and Accolades ........................ 9

The Truth About Scars............................ 15

Preventing Scars ................................. 23

The Meridian Chart .............................. 29

Alarm Points .................................... 37

Emotional Roadblocks to Healing .................. 41

The 5 Stressors .................................. 51

Painkillers: The Opioid Epidemic................... 59

Pain Is Your Friend .............................. 65

Brain Health .................................... 75

Mental Health................................... 85

Nutrition Response Testing®. . . . . . . . . . . . . . . . . . . . . . . 89

Blocks and Switches . . . . . . . . . . . . . . . . . . . . . . . . . . . . 95

NOW: Nutrition, Oxygen, and Water . . . . . . . . . . . . . . . 99

Harrower's Chart: How the Endocrine System Works. . 107

The Body as a Whole: Mind, Body, and Soul. . . . . . . . . 111

Faith and Encouragement. . . . . . . . . . . . . . . . . . . . . . . . 115

About Shannon Eggleston . . . . . . . . . . . . . . . . . . . . . . . 121

BONUS. . . . . . . . . . . . . . . . . . . . . . . . . . . . . . . . . . . . . . 123

Book Shannon to Speak . . . . . . . . . . . . . . . . . . . . . . . . . 125

Connect with Shannon . . . . . . . . . . . . . . . . . . . . . . . . . . 127

I'd Love to Hear From You. . . . . . . . . . . . . . . . . . . . . . . 129

# INTRODUCTION: WELCOME TO *THE TRUTH ABOUT SCARS AND ROADBLOCKS TO HEALING!*

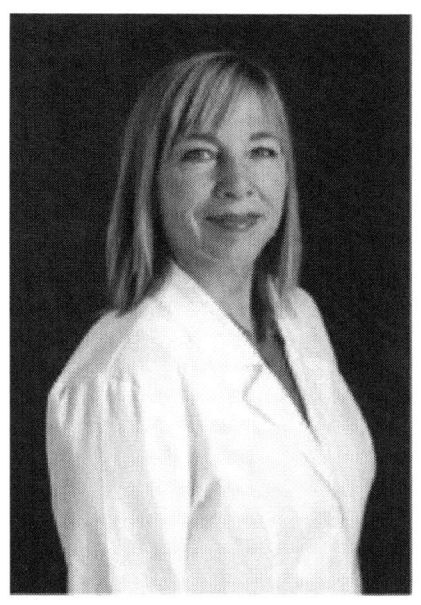

**Shannon Eggleston, Naturopath, Holistic Health Practitioner (HHP)**

Hi, my name is Shannon Eggleston. I help people heal themselves naturally and permanently so they can live pain-free and symptom-free. This book will educate you on how to recognize and overcome roadblocks to healing and get to the root cause of your symptoms.

People always ask me how I got into natural medicine. I can say my understanding of natural medicine started with growing up in Hawaii! Clean air, water, and great food were all important parts of my life. My mother was sure that if I had a problem, I was either dehydrated, exhausted, or hungry. She was right! We paddled outrigger canoes, surfed mornings and afternoons, swam, and ran a mile every day.

Aunti Pocho Kanuha was a senior canoe paddler with Kai 'Opua Outrigger Canoe Club. As my mentor, she taught me how to eat well to feel stronger. She is a great role model with plenty of energy to this day!

Aunti Pocho's brother, Jerome Kanuha, was my paddling coach. When the Ironman race came to town, he made friends with the athletes to learn their tricks for winning. He learned that one of the integral parts of winning had to do with diet and nutrition. Jerome knew we already had the training down, so he was very excited to implement this new way of eating. He learned how to fast off of carbs during the week. On race day, we would carb load early in the morning, and it was amazing how much easier it was to win! It was a game changer.

It was normal for one of the coaches to come up and push on the pressure points on my back just before the race started. Like acupressure points, when someone squeezes your shoulder, it alleviates pain and muscle stiffness. Immediately, the pain and stiffness from working out so hard left, and I felt like liquid gold when I got into the canoe. It helped me understand the power of using pressure points to relieve pain. This, along with going off of carbs the week prior, contributed to us always winning gold medals.

Years later, my mother became very ill with stomach and adrenal cancer and had to go to the hospital on the mainland. She was in terrible pain and ended up passing away without anyone using Chinese Medicine to assist in her healing. I expected Mr. Miyagi to come in and use pressure points on my mother to relieve her pain and help her heal but, alas, there was no one like a Mr. Miyagi practicing Chinese Medicine at the hospital.

As a result of this experience, I decided to go to holistic health college to be able to help others like my mother. Thank God for Mueller College in San Diego. I found my niche! Traditional Chinese Medicine made sense to me. It is a system. You can read the body like a book! I memorized lists of foods to eat when you were well or weak, and I was blessed to go to China to study. It was amazing, and it was the first time I saw any form of muscle testing being done.

After studying at the hospital in China, I understood the bridge between Western and Eastern medicine. They are so complementary; it is amazing how well they go together. Acupuncture can provide pain relief for surgery. While I was in China, I saw a picture of a surgery being performed without painkillers, using clamps on the open abdomen. The patient was wide awake without pain. The clamps to open the abdomen were placed strategically on acupuncture points to numb the area.

At Guang An Men Hospital, it was normal to be assessed and treated with deep massage and chiropractic therapy for the first six weeks of treatment. If you did not heal completely, then you would have surgery and physical therapy. All services were provided by the same doctor. He did not get paid until you were healed. One of the doctors who was training us was very proud to explain that their system healed 70% of their patients within the first six weeks using massage and chiropractic therapy, leaving only 30% that had to have surgery.

I noticed that in China, people ate very well and exercised every day. That was a long time ago in 1990. Guang An Men Hospital was a traditional teaching hospital. All of the doctors practiced an exercise called Chi Gong every morning before they started work. Chi Gong keeps the body calm and strong.

The pharmacy there used herbs as medicine exclusively. The treating doctor would give the list of symptoms to the pharmacist, who would then make a compound of medicine made out of herbs specific for that patient.

After studying in China, I settled into a private practice for about eight years and then had a chance to study nutrition with Standard Process. Nutrition made on an organic farm—what a joy! The farm is in Wisconsin and has soil very rich in nutrients. The founder of the Standard Process farm was Dr. Royal Lee. He was an inventor and held many patents, including the timer to help planes land and trains change tracks as well as the first regulator for a car. He studied the body and nutrition and was the first doctor to create a nutrition line that can rebuild the body with all-organic whole foods from the farm. The farm still exists today and is still planting all-natural, organic foods.

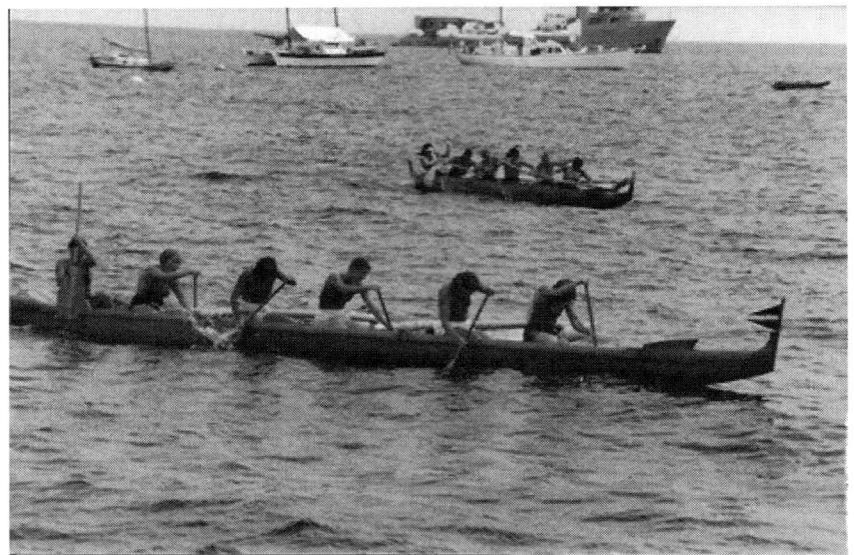

**Outrigger Canoe Paddling with Kai 'Opua Canoe Club in Kona, Hawaii. Early 1980s.**

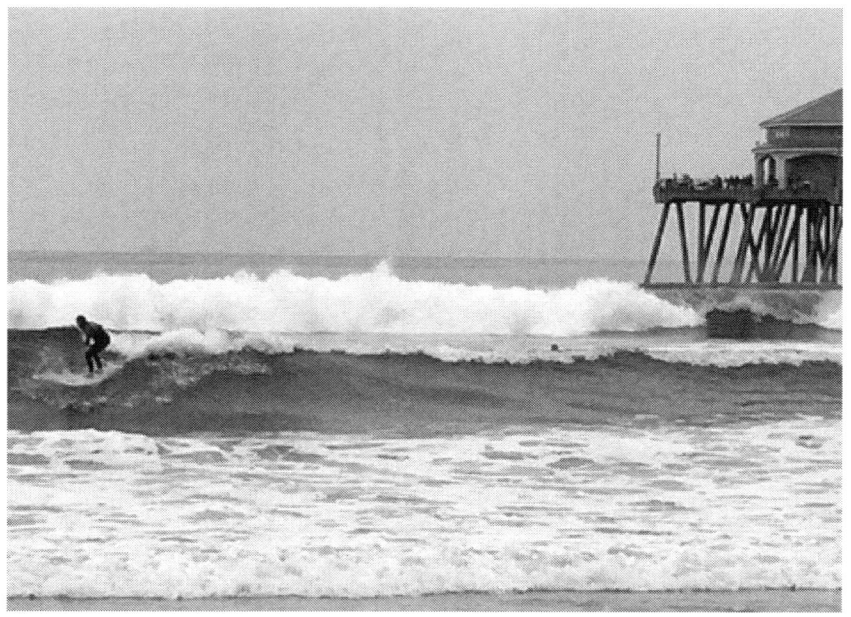

**Surfing in Huntington Beach, CA. 2017**

**Guang An Men Hospital, China 1990**

# ENDORSEMENTS AND ACCOLADES

### Proverbs 3:13 KJV
*"Happy is the man that findeth wisdom, and the man that getteth understanding."*

Thank you, God, for insisting that I write this book and for your strength and provision to see it through to those who will benefit from it. A million thanks!

**Thank you to the following for being part of that provision:**

MichelJoy DelRe, a great business coach.

My mother, for raising us without chemicals.

Evelynn Molina, for recognizing God's path for me and guiding me straight into holistic health college.

Ramona Moody, for your genius ability to teach Chinese Medicine and lead a class to the hospital and back safely and then inviting the doctors to come teach here! I love your opinions to this day.

My Father, for using his gifts to partner with the City of Hope.

The City of Hope Hospital in Duarte, for creating a safe place to study, create, and heal.

Debra and Joe Schmidt, for giving me roots, wings and ohana.

My entire family: the Egglestons, Woods, Knowles, Griffins, Schmidts, and Sarnis. You are my village.

Michael Eggleston, you and Deb were my first healing team! Mahalos for sharing all your ohana and support!

Dr. Leo Huddleston and Dr. Michael Wells, you guys are the best study partners ever thank you for all of your brilliance going through the Advanced Clinical Training at Ulan Nutritional Systems.

Dr. Ulan, Dr. Bryman, and Dr. Pulskar, for teaching me the joyful obligation of Nutrition Response Testing® and creating a network of health professionals that is highly effective and ethical as a team.

Dr. Charles Dubois, President of Standard Process Inc., for your standard of excellence in everything you do. A special shoutout to Christine Mason and her team that manages the farm. Thank you for loving what you do. And to Greg Curtis, for your passion to make each practitioner better in his or her own right in order to serve more people.

Dr. Becky Ettinger, for using your gifts to further the kingdom of God and being a great friend of Jesus and I.

Dr. Terry Rogers, my classmate, friend and mentor in Chinese Medicine.

Dr. Koakane Green, mahalo. Dr. and Mrs. Joe Teff, Dr. Vanessa Teff, Dr. Cooper, Dr. April Brunetti, Dr. Susan Bobek, Dr. Amir, Ted Flittner, Dr. Jay Robbins, Dr. Wally Schmidt, Tom Van Dyk, Diane Eggleston, and Ron Morrison, thank you all for your constant love.

Renee Ascencio, for your outstanding work ethic and your leap of faith!

I will always be grateful for my first Nutrition Response Testing® seminar with Dr. Freddie and Mrs. Dana Ulan in partnership with Dr. Robert and Lisa Curry. I appreciated the kind, professional education so much that I have kept at it for 17 years and am still going thanks to God and your gifts.

*What Our Clients Say:*

*"During 2014, I was constantly ill. Doctors could only offer maintenence antibiotics, which made me even sicker. At the end of 2014, I went to the Natural Healing Center. I immediately started to heal and become healthy again. I'm medication-free, 30 pounds lighter, healthy, energetic, and very happy."* - Cam N.

*"Fifteen years ago, I was hit by a drunk driver, instantly catapulting me into a life of near constant migraines that first year. For the next three years, I had migraines three to five days a week, and then they 'settled down' to about two to three days a week. About five years ago, I went off of gluten, and that helped some. Then, I went to Shannon three years ago, feeling very tired with lots of brain fog and depressed that I still had so many migraines.*

*The first day there, she diagnosed me with several other major food allergies (not caught in the traditional allergist's office where I had been receiving shots for two years) that I did not know I had. After a month of detoxing these out of my intestines/body, I started feeling fantastic! The brain fog was gone, the migraines had plummeted, the joint pain was much less intense, my stomach and gut did not hurt at all any longer, and I just felt so much stronger, energetic, and healthier!*

*I just turned 50 this year, yet I am not depressed about this fact since today, I feel so much better than I did in my 30s after that car accident! Shannon has been such a blessing in my life and that of my family, as they now have the real me back."* –Robin

*"I was swimming a 6:30 500M, and now I'm down to a 6:00! I feel stronger and have more stamina and energy!"* –John B.

*"I've become a very big fan! Skin and digestive problems that I've had since college (23 years ago) began to clear up in less than a week of working with Shannon Eggleston, ND. I'm even a holistic health coach, and I regularly help others heal themselves, but I was not able to heal myself (despite the best nutrition, herbs, organic foods, and many integrative health practitioners). In my first session, she clearly saw what*

*was a priority for my body, then gave me clear instructions on how to help my body naturally repair itself. I'm so, SO grateful! Since I started seeing her three weeks ago, I've noticed that I sleep way better, my skin is clearing up, I'm having healthy bowel movements, I have more energy, I'm thinking clearer, and I no longer wake up with a tight/sore back. Also, I've noticed that I'm feeling more optimistic about my health, which makes me more optimistic about my future, which is giving me more peace! This is the real deal, folks."* –Press M.

*"Prior to going to the Natural Healing Center, I was tired, stressed, and exhausted* all *the time. I am now much more calm, stable, and energized. I continue to go to maintain my newfound endurance and energy for cycling!"* –Richard M.

# THE TRUTH ABOUT SCARS

**Proverbs 1:5 ESV**
*"Let the wise hear and increase in learning,
and the one who understands obtain guidance."*

Scars! It is important to find out if you have any scars on your skin (including your scalp and in your mouth) that are active. If they are active, they can cause your nervous system to malfunction.

I have been observing scars and their effects on the nervous system for over 20 years. Scars can make your heart rate increase without regulation, interrupt your sleeping, cause you to wake up many times in one night, ruin your digestion, and more. Sometimes, they can even impair your hearing, vision, and flexibility.

Oh yes… Scars can also throw a wrench in your weight loss or weight gain goals.

Your skin is your largest organ, and if you don't take care of it, it can cause a lot of problems. We take our skin for granted because we can see that it heals on the outside, but what we don't know is that it is not always completely healed the way that the body wants it to be healed. Unbeknownst to us, our body has its own ideas of what is "completely healed."

Active scars on the body can cause interference to the communication pathways from organs to the brain. It is estimated that about 80 percent of our sympathetic nerve fibers are in the skin. When these scars are acting as a roadblock to these communication pathways, it stops all functions of the pathway blocking the flow of energy which affects your circulation and oxygenation of your tissues. For example, think of an overturned semi truck backing up all lanes of a freeway. Health can be adversely affected by causing interference to proper functioning.

The meridian system is the freeway of our body. When scars cross a meridian or lie along its course, the scar impacts the electrical flow throughout that meridian. Even small scars (especially around the midline of the body) can have a serious effect. C-section, episiotomy, circumcision and vasectomy scars, and even the navel are examples of scars on the midline of the body.

Holes in the body such as pierced navels, nose rings, pierced ears, and tongue rings are scars. Navel rings almost always have a negative effect, as they not only cross and disrupt the energy flow, but also because they are metal, which means they can have an electromagnetic effect. Usually, this jewelry must be removed, and the piercing should be treated as a scar. Tattoos, stretch marks, and burns can also have this effect.

The adrenal glands are the security guards of the body. As the security guards, it is their job to release adrenaline in a dangerous situation. This occurs to give us the ability to react to the situation by making us stronger and faster. Adrenaline is only meant to be released in dangerous situations so we have quick reflexes. For example, if you have to jump out of the way of a falling tree, adrenaline would give you the ability to move quickly.

When the adrenal glands release adrenaline, it stops the formation of stomach acid. Without stomach acid, there is no digestion and, therefore, we don't break down our food and get the nutrition from it. If we don't get the nutrition, our bodies malfunction and break down.

Unfortunately, even if we only have a cat scratch or a papercut, the adrenal glands still react the same as if it were a dangerous situation. When the adrenals get the information that the skin has a scratch, it immediately causes an elevated release of adrenaline. Therefore, it is important to put a wound treatment on as soon as possible to secure the area. In turn, this action sends a message to the adrenals that we are not in a dangerous situation. It is important to keep the wound covered until it is not active anymore (i.e., no scab, completely healed over, and no redness).

Some scars are white while others are red or purple. As a scar heals, it will turn colors and then become skin color again or close to it. Even old scars can usually become the color of our normal skin again. It is critical to rub your scars until they become deactivated.

The process that I describe is the easiest, probably the

most affordable, and sometimes the only way to get your body to calm down enough to heal. Whether it is ringing in your ears or a back ache that just won't stop, sometimes, the only remedy that will work is rubbing your scars with organic sesame seed oil for four minutes each in the morning and before bedtime.

Some scars act crazy by sucking your healing energy up because they want to heal. So when they are treated, you can feel strange fireworks tingling all over your body. Don't worry. Slow down and keep breathing. You have just experienced stored energy being released. It will pass! Then, be sure to stretch out where you felt the fireworks/tingling/electrical zinging. Stretch that area for 45 seconds while breathing peacefully without pain or discomfort.

If the scar is too tender to massage, just lay your hand on it and breathe. Breathe in the good healing oxygen, and breathe out the pain. Once the scar is less tender, it is then ready for treatment.

## HOW TO RUB SCARS AWAY FOR FAST-TRACK HEALING:

- Rub scars gently and slowly with the organic oil your body chooses (wheat germ oil, organic sesame oil, or organic black currant seed oil) two times a day, in the morning and at bedtime, for four minutes each. You can purchase high-quality organic oils from Standard Process.

### THE TRUTH ABOUT SCARS 19

- If your scar is horizontal, rub vertically.

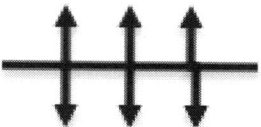

- If your scar is vertical, rub horizontally.

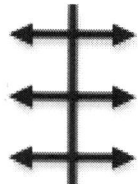

- If the scar is a circle, rub around and back and forth.

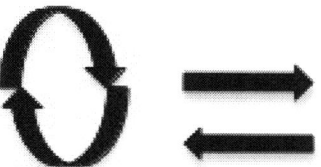

- If you have a lot of scars, it's okay to only rub half of your scars at a time. Make a list of them, then divide your body down the center (head to foot) and do the right side one time and the left side the next time.

- Testing shows it's best to massage oil into your scars before you shower.

Chinese cupping and cold laser therapy are two additional treatments for scars. Chinese cupping therapy is a favorite for helping keloid scars to flatten out. A cold laser is a high-intensity light (or energy) that operates at a specific frequency to increase healing to the scar area. The increased oxygen is used by the cells to facilitate the repair of the injured tissue. A four- to five-minute application of the cold laser to the scar may need to be repeated every other day until healing is complete.

It is estimated that high-quality oils and massage will handle 90 percent of scar problems. Adding in cupping and cold laser therapy will take it to 95 percent. And the two applications combined will handle about 98 percent of scars. The remaining 2 percent need further evaluation and treatment by an advanced Nutrition Response Testing® clinician. In a small number of cases, neural therapy may be necessary. This therapy injects the scar with a healing substance by needle.

If you want extra healing for your scars, castor oil packs are an old-fashioned remedy that everyone should know about. Cut a piece of wool or flannel to fit the scar, saturate the cloth with castor oil, and cover it with plastic wrap or something tight to keep it next to your body overnight. Wear old clothes and lay a towel down on your bedding so the oil doesn't ruin it.

My personal testimonial to castor oil is that I lacerated my eyebrow wide open in a surfing accident. Upon getting home after receiving stitches, I put on colloidal silver and a

3M waterproof bandage, then applied the castor oil pack and wrapping. By morning, my black eye was gone!

*What Our Clients Say:*

*"If you have a C-section, you must see Dr. Shannon, as she does a state-of-the-art scar therapy. I could not imagine my life without her treatment. She is very welcoming and friendly. Eight weeks after my C-section, I felt like I had a rock at the site of the surgery even though the doctor told me I was healed and ready to hit the gym. Dr. Shannon's treatment helped my scar heal and made me pain-free. She follows up very well with her patients."* –Aloma B.

*"When I started to rub my scars, I immediately felt more relaxed in my body and slept peacefully. Also, I experienced longer periods of sleep. Even if I had to get up for the bathroom, I fell right back to sleep."* – Jake C.

*"I rubbed my scars with sesame seed oil, and my headache went away. I was very surprised!"* –Adrian M.

# PREVENTING SCARS

*"An ounce of prevention is worth a pound of cure."*
Benjamin Franklin

## Prevention Is Key: Proper Wound Care Prevents Scars

The first choice for proper wound care is colloidal silver 500 PPM (part per million). Colloidal silver contains 99.99% pure silver particles suspended indefinitely in demineralized water that kills bacteria and viruses. The presence of colloidal silver near a virus, fungi, bacteria or any other single celled pathogen disables its oxygen-metabolism enzyme.

Place it directly on the wound and the surrounding area everywhere a bandage will touch. Air dry. Apply a 3M waterproof bandage. The area is now secure under that bandage. It is waterproof, so it can go surfing or in the shower or bathtub. It likes to stay on for at least five to 10 days. I do not even attempt to take them off unless the edges are frayed.

Also, other products I trust very much are grape and grapefruit seed extracts. They are antibiotic, antiviral, and anti-fungal like colloidal silver 500 PPM.

Both of these products work well. I have found that colloidal silver allows the bandage to stick better because the grapefruit seed extract by nature has some oil in it. The waterproof 3M bandage comes in a lot of different varieties. My favorite is called Tegaderm because it is big, and I can cut it to size. They also come in a box like regular bandages in three different sizes. (For your entertainment, some of them even have pictures on them.)

**THE BOX MUST SAY "3M WATERPROOF" TO KEEP YOUR WOUND SECURED.**

Everyone is different, and some skin cannot handle adhesives. In that situation, I would use non-stick pads and then use gauze to wrap around the area and secure the bandage. You should change it twice daily and use colloidal silver 500 PPM each time.

Remember that proper wound care means fewer scars. Using these methods, I have avoided scars 99 percent of the time.

**DO SCARS EVER POSE A PROBLEM IN THE FUTURE?**

Yes, it is possible that they can become "active" again after months or years and may need some additional attention. This is another reason why periodically getting your nutrition checked makes perfect sense. That way, you can catch potential issues before they affect your health.

**TIP:**

**Stock your First Aid Kit with 3M waterproof bandages and a bottle of Colloidal Silver 500 ppm**

# THE MERIDIAN CHART

**Proverbs 4:7 KJV**
*"Wisdom is the principal thing; therefore get wisdom: and with all thy getting get understanding."*

28  SCARS AND ROADBLOCKS TO HEALING

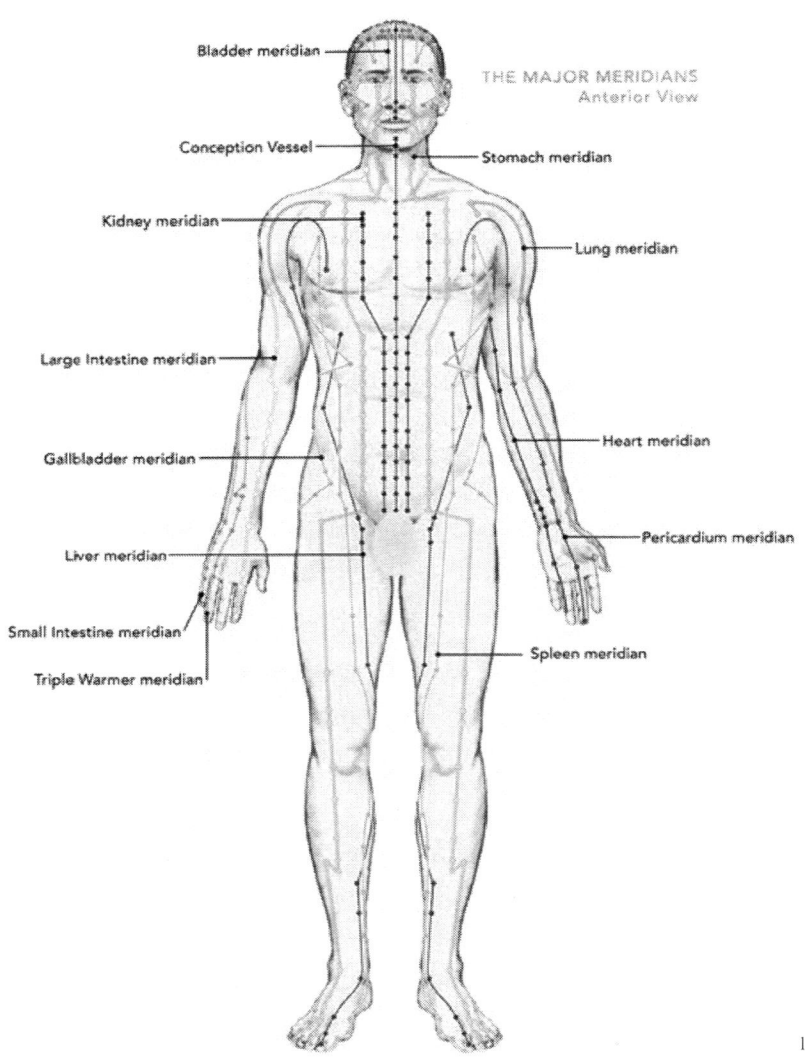

The meridian chart is derived from Traditional Chinese Medicine. It shows 12 regular meridian lines on the skin going up and down the body that are all connected and flow endlessly in a closed circuit. This system

---

1. Shen-Nong, Traditional Chinese Medicine, http://www.shen-nong.com. Retrieved February 21, 2018.

is identical on the right and left sides of the body. There are two independent meridian lines on the midline of the body that keep the body's core strong inside and out. They are seen here as the Conception Vessel, known in Chinese Medicine as the Du and Ren meridians.

In Traditional Chinese Medicine, there is something known as the life force, otherwise known as chi in Chinese. These pathways allow energy to run continuously and strengthen the body like an electrical force field. This force field also strengthens the inner organs. Each meridian carries the name of its matching organ. The meridians represent the following organs in succession:

| | |
|---|---|
| Stomach | Pericardium (Circulation) |
| Spleen | Sanjiao – Emotional Heart (Triple Warmer) |
| Heart | Gallbladder |
| Small Intestine | Liver |
| Bladder | Lung |
| Kidney | Large Intestine |

Eggleston, Shannon 2017, Meridian Chart

When the electricity runs through the meridian, it strengthens the organ it is named for. Likewise, if there is a scar on the meridian pathway, it will weaken the internal organ as well. The meridian pathways are connected end-to-end. It is a closed circuit, and, therefore, a dysfunction in one will affect the other because they are end to end.

Knowing this helps us to understand the importance of having the meridians of energy running freely at all times, enhancing the strength of the body inside and out. Each side of the body and the midline can be shut down completely by an active scar or wound. Just like traffic backing up when there is a semi truck overturned on the freeway, if there is a scar on one meridian, the entire circuit stops flowing. The energy then piles up into the scar and does not continue on its pathway.

The scar does not know it is healed, so it keeps taking the electricity to heal itself. The active scar absorbs the electricity into itself so much that there is no more electricity to continue on the pathway of the circuit. By treating the scar, it will stop absorbing the electricity of the force field for eight hours.

Most times, you can rub the scar with organic sesame seed oil for four minutes twice a day, and this will allow the force field to run unhindered and strengthen the body again. There are other meridians, and understanding of all of them is as important in Traditional Chinese Medicine as understanding the anatomy in Western medicine.

We use Traditional Chinese Medicine to ascertain what is needed for healing and when. Each organ heals at a specific time every two hours of the day and night. Knowing what time the organs go into healing mode helps us to know what time of day to get the appropriate nutrients for the body to heal that specific organ.

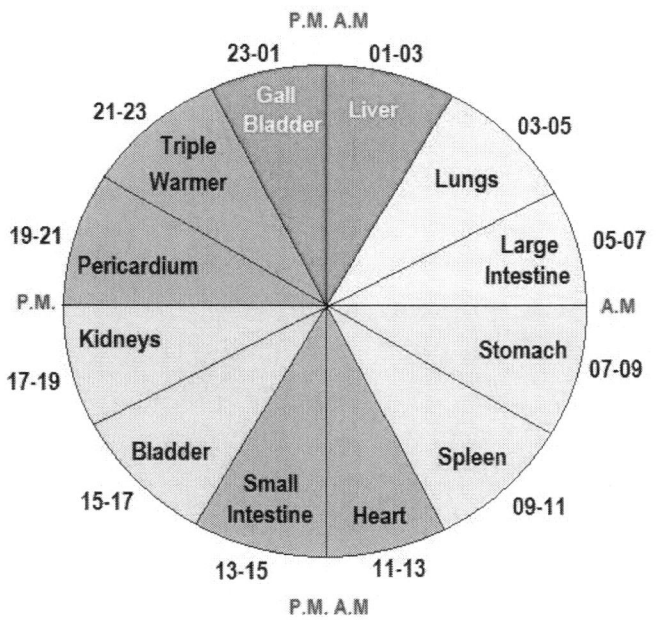

**Chinese Meridian Body Clock**

The lungs heal from 3 a.m. to 5 a.m. Lungs are part of your filter system. To function optimally, the lungs must have a clean diet, clean water, and a happy heart. In times of grief, the lungs are affected the most. Deep grieving can

---

2. Chinese Body Clock, http://www.spiritualcoach.com/chinese-body-clock/ (Retrieved March 7, 2018)

make the lungs weak. So if you find yourself sad or grieving, the best remedy is to take action! Cheer someone up to make them feel better. By doing this, you will feel better too. Take a walk out in nature, and take the time to really appreciate everything for its beauty. Other things you may consider are exercising, making a list of everything you are thankful and grateful for, writing a letter to someone you love and haven't seen in a long time, dancing, drawing, or painting. Do something you enjoy! Be sure to share your grief with someone you love so that you feel heard and connected. You can also give your grief to Jesus and feel better immediately. Life force flows from the lungs to the large intestine.

The large intestine heals in the morning between 5 a.m. to 7 a.m. To heal, it needs to be cleaned. It needs plenty of lettuce and green leafy vegetables, other vegetables, raw olives, clean water, and good raw nuts and seeds to clean itself and function. Life force flows from the large intestine meridian into the stomach meridian.

The stomach heals from 7 a.m. to 9 a.m. It's good to have breakfast before 9 a.m. since that is when the stomach is healing and calming. When you experience anxiety, your stomach doesn't function well. If you are under enough stress, the adrenals release adrenaline throughout the body, preparing the body to fight or run from danger. When you are fighting or running from danger, there is no time to sit and eat. Remember to sit down, chew your food thoroughly, and try to calmly focus on only one thing: digesting your food. Enjoy it peacefully and gratefully. Your digestion starts here. Chewing thoroughly allows the food to mix with saliva and begin the digestion process. That way, when it gets to the stomach, stomach acid can break it down and continue the digestion process properly. The body's life force flows from the stomach meridian into the spleen meridian.

The spleen heals from 9 a.m. to 11 a.m. The spleen is a very big part of your immune system and is located underneath your left ribs. If you eat too much sugar, you could make your bottom left ribs hurt. The less sugar and dessert you eat, the better off your spleen is. The spleen also makes red blood cells. To make your spleen happy, leave onions around your house and office. Onions absorb bacteria, viruses, and fungus. Leave them out with the skin on. It doesn't matter what color they are, but the bigger, the better. The spleen meridian life force flows into the heart meridian.

The heart heals between 11 a.m. and 1 p.m. The heart holds the spirit and its essence. The heart is guarded by the thyroid and the adrenals. When the thyroid is unregulated, the heart is at risk because there is nothing governing the regulation of your heart rate (i.e., thyroid, adrenals, pituitary). The life force flows from the heart meridian into small intestine meridian.

The small intestine heals between the hours of 1 p.m. and 3 p.m. The small intestine meridian is what you use to activate or sedate the heart for Jet Lag Reduction Therapy, which I will explain at the end of this book. The life force flows from the small intestine meridian into the bladder meridian.

The bladder heals from 3 p.m. to 5 p.m. It must have plenty of fresh water. Half your body weight in ounces is usually enough. Sometimes, your body will need more for healing or detoxing. A good example of perfect water is rain water from a well that has no toxins in it or unpolluted spring water. If you do not drink enough water, the body gets tired and droopy in the afternoon between 3 p.m. and 5 p.m. Water is better at energizing the body than caffeine. Drink water to avoid the afternoon slump and immediately feel stronger. A solid 12 ounces or more works great. Life force flows from the bladder meridian into the kidney meridian.

The kidneys heal from 5 p.m. to 7 p.m. Oftentimes, when there is kidney pain, it is because the drain pipe between the kidney and bladder is blocked by a silty sludge of some kind and needs to be cleaned out. It's amazing how well the kidneys can work when the ureter is clean. The life force flows from the kidney meridian into the pericardium meridian.

The pericardium heals between 7 p.m. and 9 p.m. The pericardium protects and guards over the spirit and the heart. Life force flows from the pericardium into the sanjiao — emotional heart (TW).

The sanjiao — emotional heart (TW) heals between 9 p.m. and 11 p.m. Being emotionally upset or overly excited (as in spending all day at Disneyland) can cause emotional exhaustion, indigestion, vomiting, diarrhea, edema, pain, and stiffness in the lower back. Life force flows from the sanjiao – emotional heart (TW) meridian into the gall bladder meridian.

The gallbladder heals between 11 p.m. and 1 a.m. If there are too many hot fats, fried foods, or hot spices in your diet that disrupt your digestive process, it will be difficult to sleep during this time. Also, being agitated can make sleep difficult during this time. The life force flows from the gallbladder meridian into the liver meridian.

The liver heals from 1 a.m. to 3 a.m. There are many jobs for the liver to do. Without getting too complicated, suffice it to say that too much caffeine and sugar can keep you awake during this time or wake you up if you have fallen asleep.

It's also important to note that your blood sugar must be regulated to sleep well through the night. If you drink too much wine or eat too much dessert, you might not sleep through the night, as sugar is a stimulant. If you have too much sugar at night, it causes a blood sugar low (as in a sugar crash), and your body wakes up. By the same token, if you don't eat enough food, then you'll also have a blood sugar low, and your body may wake up at night because it's hungry. Your body needs sustenance to make it through the night.

The body makes its own sugar out of nutritious food. If you eat processed sugar, your body cannot use it. Processed sugar breaks down cell walls, causing your body to deteriorate. Processed sugar is in almost everything except whole foods. By eating whole foods, your body can make its own sugar to create cells properly.

Deep anger can also show up as a toxin in the liver. I have seen people give their anger to God, back off the caffeine, sugar, and fried foods, and be able to sleep through the night when nothing else has worked. We have a prayer ministry to help with deep-seated anger, and we ask our Father God to show us who we are angry at so we can forgive them and let go of our anger. Only our Father God knows the truth of our hearts. The liver works easier without being weighed down by hatred. The life force flows from the liver meridian into the lung meridian to complete the circuit.

The Chinese Meridian Body Clock explains when each organ heals. If you are having any problems during these times, it means the body clock is not running smoothly, as the electricity is supposed to run through each meridian. When there is an emotional or physical block, the flow of chi stops in one meridian and piles up in the other, making all of the organs get out of balance.

# ALARM POINTS

**Proverbs 8:11 KJV**
*"For wisdom is better than rubies; and all the things that may be desired are not to be compared to it."*

Alarm points tell you if something is seriously wrong. My Aunt Ellie went to every doctor that money could buy for two years, telling them that she had a stabbing pain in her side. They would run tests yet find nothing. They would tell her to go home, as she was just having pain because she was a woman. Had anyone known the alarm points of Traditional Chinese Medicine, my aunt would not have had to suffer for two years in pain before her liver cancer was diagnosed.

When an alarm point is active, it is a hot, piercing pain. It can hurt as if someone is stabbing you. It is part of the body's warning system, and knowing the alarm points can save your life two years ahead of time.

# 38　SCARS AND ROADBLOCKS TO HEALING

Below is a chart of the body's alarm points ([3]):

- Lung
- Circulation sex
- Heart
- Stomach
- Liver
- Gallbladder
- Large intestine
- Triple warmer
- Small intestine
- Bladder
- Spleen
- Kidney

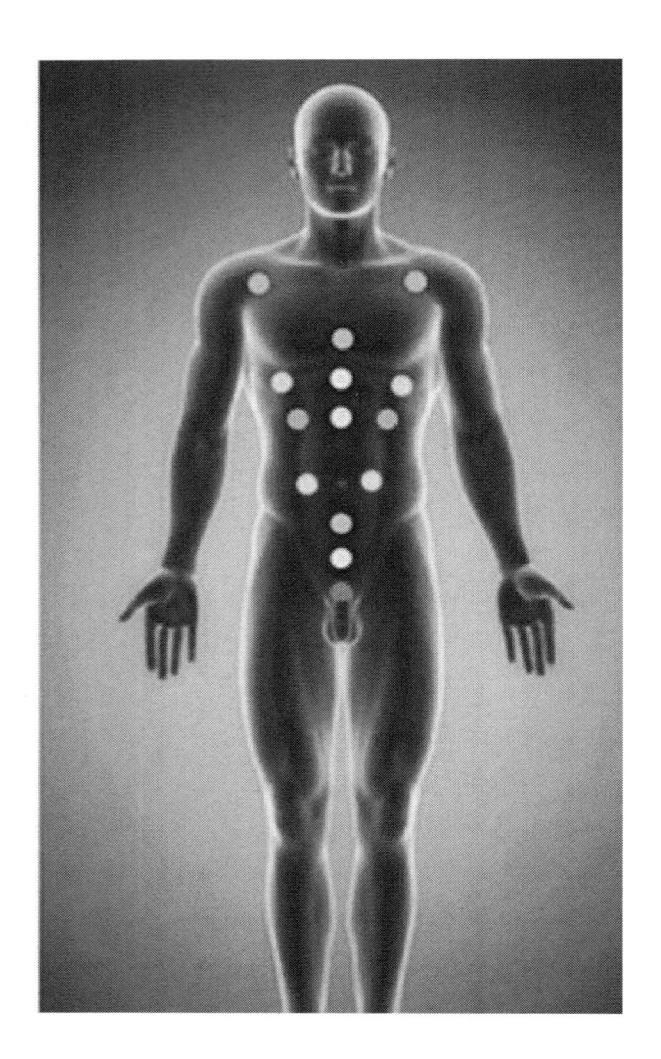

Alarm points are all along the midline torso. Four on each side and six on the midline. To relieve pain, hold the active

---

3. Rita Rooks, http://attunedmasterenergyhealing.com/2015/07/12/to-activate-your-chi-energy-easily-everyday/. Retrieved February 26, 2018.

alarm point gently and breathe the pain out. As the pain dissipates, press harder. Do this technique while breathing cool air in and exhaling the pain repeatedly until the pain is gone. Breathing deeply and peacefully works well. After the pain lessens, check it every day to make sure it stays clear.

If the alarm point is active and the pain cannot be alleviated by breath, then it is important to do what is necessary to immediately alleviate the pain. Address all stressors. The worst offenders should be the first to leave. Get rid of sodas, processed foods, and caffeine of any kind. You should also give up sugar of any kind, including cookies, cakes, candies, and ice cream. It is important to eat good, clean, green vegetables.

It is important to handle an alarm point immediately. Do not ignore an alarm point. It is the body's way of sounding an alarm before the damage is done.

---

**If you have pain on an alarm point, let's find out what it is as soon as possible.**

**Call (877) 953-3869 or visit**

**http://naturalhealingcenter.us/contact**

# EMOTIONAL ROADBLOCKS TO HEALING

**Proverbs 4:23 NIV**
*"Above all else, guard your heart,
for everything you do flows from it."*

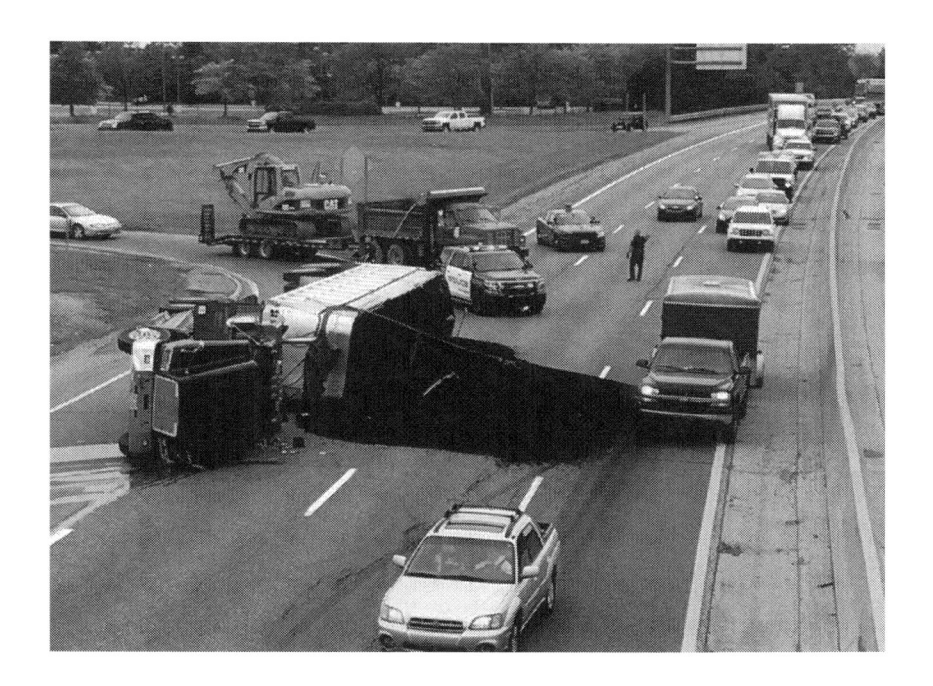

A nything that can keep you from healing would be considered a roadblock.

Emotional blocks to healing are huge and can look like sabotage eating or poor eating habits, bad self talk, saying bad things about yourself, repeating what other people say that is bad about you, etc.

Yes, emotional scars can hold you back from being your complete self! A good example is arthritis. People with arthritis markers have some things in common. The emotional side of arthritis is inherited from our parents and grandparents as well as those we grew up around. We mimic what we hear growing up. For example, when our parents talk negatively about themselves and make fun of themselves, we do too. Bad self talk can create pain and disease.

The first time I heard this, I was in China, studying at a hospital. I asked the head Chinese doctor to teach me how to treat people with arthritis. He resoundingly responded, "No, no, no! I don't want to talk about arthritis!" I said, "Please- it's for my family! He was exasperated and asked me why I wanted to know how to treat arthritis. He said, "People who have arthritis that comes and goes have to be taught how to think better, and this is very difficult to teach. Thinking poorly, saying bad things about yourself all day, and agreeing with negative people is not good."

Every time I have met a person with rheumatoid arthritis, I have confirmed that they inherited the way they think bad thoughts from their parents and/or their grandparents. People who have successfully had arthritis and go into remission have learned how to eat better, speak better, and make better choices for the good of their bodies and souls.

Inheriting bad thinking patterns is very simple since we learn everything from our parents and the world around us. It is easy to understand how insignificant these things can seem. A good example of this would be how a father tells his child, "Come on, let's go! You are as slow as a snail and such a pain in my butt." Even though the father says this jokingly and with love, the child takes it as truth. Now, when that young man grows up and has his own children, he says the same thing to his child, only usually not so nicely. Either way, the child knows the story that he is slow and a pain in the butt.

Children are impressionable and happy to pattern everything to be a good child. If a child is born to an angry, bitter person, that child will show anger and bitter attitudes to be acceptable to the parent and to fit in. On the other hand, a peaceful child brought up with encouragement, love, and good speaking patterns about themselves and others grows up that way and continues the inheritance for their children.

Dr. Caroline Leaf is a cognitive neuroscientist with a PhD in Communication Pathology and a BSc in Logopedics and Audiology, specializing in metacognitive and cognitive neuropsychology. She is from Australia, and she wrote a book entitled *Switch on Your Brain*. It shows the deterioration of the brain when you speak negatively and how prayer rebuilds the brain.

According to her research, the vast majority-a whopping 75 to 98 percent-of the illnesses that plague us today are a direct result of our thought life. What we think about truly affects us both physically and emotionally. In fact, fear alone triggers more than 1,400 known physical and chemical responses in our bodies, activating more than thirty different hormones! Today, our culture is undergoing an epidemic of toxic thoughts that, when left unchecked, create ideal conditions for illnesses.

Dr. Masaru Emoto, the Japanese scientist, revolutionized the idea that our thoughts and intentions impact the physical realm. He is one of the most important water researchers the world has known. He proved that by speaking over water, it changes the molecules positively or negatively. When we speak negatively, it creates negative reactions in our blood and tissue. When we speak positively, as in prayer, our bodies heal. There are pictures from his book online showing water molecules. When he speaks the word "love" over them, they look like beautiful snowflakes. Then, when he says the word "peace" over the molecules, they change to other beautiful snowflakes. When he says the word "anger," the molecules turn black!

That knowledge, along with the information that the Chinese doctor gave me, is substantial proof that self talk really can change the way your blood responds because blood is made up of water as a base. It can either heal or kill.

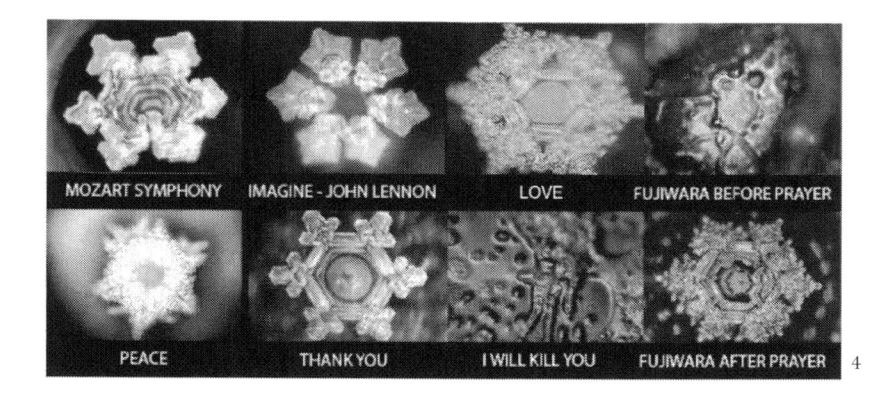

| MOZART SYMPHONY | IMAGINE - JOHN LENNON | LOVE | FUJIWARA BEFORE PRAYER |
| PEACE | THANK YOU | I WILL KILL YOU | FUJIWARA AFTER PRAYER |[4]

Other books that explain this are the Bible and the *The 7 Habits of Successful People* by Stephen R. Covey. Choose peace and love for yourself. Practice saying encouraging words to yourself. For example, try saying, "Good job," "it's going to be OK," "you can do it," and "this too shall pass." By choosing peace, your central nervous system will reflect peace. You can practice deep, peaceful breathing anywhere to calm down—even on the freeway! Breathing deeply can change a stressful moment into an acceptable moment, thereby relieving stomach tension, neck tension, and a host of other problems. Peaceful people usually do not have disease.

When you sing something that makes your heart happy, your body works better as a machine. One example of this is was a doctor who just could not bear to tell his terminally ill patients that they were going to die. So, with all the love in his heart, he would look into their eyes and say, "Well, all we have left is a song and a prayer."

---

4. Masaru Emoto, 2010, http://www.masaru-emoto.net/english/water-crystal.html. Retrieved February 21, 2018.

He couldn't believe his eyes when he saw one of his most terminally ill patients a year later on the street alive and walking at a nice pace. He called after her and said, "How are you? And when did you get well?" She thanked him and said, "Well, you told me all I had was a song and a prayer, so I started singing and praying, and it worked!"

Personally, I have taken that story to heart because my mother died of cancer and I don't want to duplicate that, so I've been singing and praying for a long time now (especially when I feel bad). It works great!

"If I weren't so fat, if I weren't so stupid, if only I had done it this way, if only I…"

Whatever the excuses, those words are a white flag of surrender. If I hear the words "should've," "would've," "could've," or "if only," I wave a white flag in my head and surrender to peace and say, "It's going to be alright. This is going to work out great! Not a problem." (Even if it seems like a very big problem, I tell myself otherwise, and that leaves me available to look for a solution.)

I believe there is a benevolent God who looks after us, loves us, and truly shows us a way out of problems when we read His Word, believe it, and thank Him ahead of time for helping us.

**Love yourself, and be kind to yourself.** Do what's right for your soul. Your body is listening to you.

**Bitterness, unforgiveness, anger, and sadness are all roadblocks to healing.** It is very important to deal with these internal roadblocks because they can get in the way of your physical healing. One way you know that you are bitter, angry, sad, lonely, or tired is that you will notice how you speak differently when you're upset. For example, you may speak with a sharp voice and snap at someone, justifying your reaction due to what has happened to you in the past.

**Healing is a choice of the will.** Choosing to let go of bitterness means looking ahead with a positive attitude. Everyone has problems, and most everyone has had a broken heart or been wronged by someone. There is freedom in honesty. Say the truth by sunset or as soon as you realize that you hurt someone's feelings or someone hurt your feelings. Call them and apologize. Say, "I'm sorry I hurt your feelings. I didn't mean to. Please forgive me." It is very honest to say, "Ouch, I got home and realized my feelings were hurt today when you said XYZ. It didn't work for me, and I thought you would like to know."

**By saying the truth when your feelings are hurt, two things happen.** First, you won't hold bitterness because of it. And second, it gives the person a heads-up about what has happened. I love the chance to make things right. Being honest is being loving to yourself and others. Even if the other person does not respond, you have still done the right thing by yourself. Making sure that you don't hold on to anger and bitterness and sadness will help you heal.

**Anger is okay as long as it does not cause you to do anything hurtful.** It is good if it causes you to write a letter or do something to rectify the situation. It is not good if it causes you to internalize feelings, hurt yourself, or eat foods that are bad for you. Often, the reason you are upset is not even because of what happened that day. It is because something that happened today triggered an upset in your past that never got handled or healed.

**The Bible says that we will be forgiven by God as we forgive others**. I write down everything I want to say about my hurt feelings, and then, when I am done talking about it, I say out loud to God, "I choose to forgive. Even though it caused me a lot of grief, I choose to forgive them. Thank you for helping me forgive them."

I love to get that off my chest and into God's hands so that when my brain wants to complain, I won't! The only way I know how to get rid of sadness is to give it to Jesus. He really understands sadness. Nothing else I have ever done works as well. I might be crying, but as soon as I remember, I say out loud, "Lord Jesus, I give you my sadness." Then, I imagine handing it to him as if I were handing him a letter. I take a big breath and feel relief because I am loved. You are loved too. It really works! Peace be with you as you choose to heal and be kind to yourself.

> **Consider a session of healing prayer.** Contact your church or call Natural Healing Center for an appointment; we will teach you how to talk directly to God and hear from Him. We love the way He loves and protects us in healing.
>
> **(877) 953-3869**
> or
> Visit http://naturalhealingcenter.us/contact

*Per our client:*

"Dr. Shannon is one of my favorite persons in this world! She is a very lovely, caring, upbeat, gifted by God, intuitive natural healer. She was able to find root issues in me when no one else could. I trust her and truly believe she has a genuine heart to see people get better." —Aimee S.

# THE 5 STRESSORS

*"Anything can cause anything."* –Dr. Fred Ulan

There are five stressors[5] that cause blocks to nerve pathways and can affect your healing.

1. Foods – sensitivities and allergies to certain foods
2. Heavy metal toxins – from metal fillings, aluminum in deodorant, birth control devices
3. Chemical toxins – from chlorine, hair dye, household or work chemicals, medications
4. Immune challenges – viruses, bacteria, yeast, parasites, and other organisms
5. Scar interference – large or small

Our bodies are made to clean everything out of the blood. Anything toxic that you breathe, eat, or that goes through your skin needs to be cleansed. The good news is that our bodies are made to cleanse themselves naturally. The problem is when there are too many toxins to keep up with.

---

5. Rosen, Paul J. *The Great Health Heist*, Cornelius, NC, Warren Publishing Inc., 2007.

Our bodies were not made to drink water with chemicals such as chlorine and fluoride, eat food with addicting chemicals, or breathe air polluted with lead and pesticides. In a perfect world, we would have fresh spring water, clean food from clean seeds, clean fresh air, and a safe, clean environment to live in.

Food sensitivities can make you feel like you have the flu, give you rashes, fevers, congestion, and breathing problems. It is hard to imagine how sick you can become when your body has a reaction to food as if it were poisoned.

Metal toxicity can result in the same reactions and sometimes cause food reactions. I have seen food sensitivities go away when the metal toxicity has been cleaned out. High levels of mercury, silver, lead, and nickel can be found in the tissues of people who have amalgam fillings. High levels of metals can cause severe reactions such as rashes, fatigue, nausea, ringing in the ears, and other immune challenges.

It is most necessary to use a dam when you're having mercury fillings taken out. The dam is a piece of plastic put over your mouth. Your dentist will pop the tooth he or she is working on through the plastic. This prevents the mercury from touching the skin in your mouth or down your throat. Mercury is poisonous, as it outgasses in your mouth at all times. I recommend using a biological dentist for removing mercury fillings because they are well-versed in safety measures to keep you well.

Toxic chemicals include pesticides, plastics, chlorine,

fluoride, dry cleaning chemicals, and acetates, just to name a few. It's easy to unknowingly breathe in chemicals that are toxic to the body. For example, when you're riding a bicycle, you may be exposed to pesticides. When swimming in a pool, you may breathe in chlorine. Likewise, when you're getting your hair or nails done, you are exposed to acetates and perfumes. These are all harmful airborne chemicals that get into your lungs and eyes.

We've been duped about fluoride. We have been taught that fluoride is good for our teeth, but that is not true. It causes deterioration of the teeth and bones. Learn why Sweden, Norway, Austria, Finland, China, and more countries have banned fluoride: Flouride Poison on Tap Documentary bit.ly/2LXNhLx.

Your skin is porous, and anything you put on it goes into your bloodstream, creating a toxic stress on your liver. It is best to use personal care products such as lotions, soaps, shampoos, deodorant, makeup, etc. that are free of chemicals. Chemicals in these products, as well as in our day-to-day lives include sodium lauryl sulfate, isopropyl alcohol, fluoride, aluminum, phthalates, dry cleaning chemicals such as formaldehyde, and fire retardants used in clothing, etc. For a complete list of chemicals you should avoid, I recommend going to the Environmental Working Group's site: https://www.ewg.org. Learn more about these dangerous chemicals and whether or not they are present in your current products.

These are things that we don't typically think of, but they are dangerous. It is not safe to drink water out of a plastic bottle that has been left in a hot car. Nor is it safe to eat food that has been heated up in plastic. The plastic melts, and then poisons get into the food and water. These toxins are called dioxins. Per the World Health Organization, dioxins are highly toxic and can cause reproductive and developmental problems, damage the immune system, interfere with hormones, and also cause cancer. Due to the omnipresence of dioxins, all people have background exposure, which is not expected to affect humans. However, due to the highly toxic potential, efforts need to be undertaken to reduce current background exposure.[6]

Being aware of chemical exposure can help you take precautions. Wear eye protection around chemicals. For example, you should wear sunglasses when you are walking through a smoky casino or bicycling. Go to a natural salon where they use chemical-free products. Just be aware, and take precautions.

Immune challenges are yeast, mold, bacteria, and viruses. A word to the wise: be very careful about water damage causing airborne mold spores. They can be deadly. Mold, yeast, and fungus can cause leaky gut, which can make you feel sick and weak with a lot of brain fog and even loopiness. It eats holes in your intestines, which can allow poisons from your intestines to get into your blood.

Bacteria and viruses are common. When your immunity

---

6. WHO, "Dioxins and their Effect on Human Health," http://www.who.int/mediacentre/factsheets/fs225/en/. Retrieved February 25, 2018.

is down or weakened, your body cannot easily fight them off. They are particularly common during the change of season. The constant fluctuation between hot and cold puts stress on your body and makes you tired and rundown.

By strengthening your body, you will be able to fight them off better as well as avoid illness.

There are several ways you can strengthen your body. It is imperative to ensure you are first covering the basics:

1. Get eight hours of sleep per night
2. Drink unadulterated fresh spring water (half your body weight in ounces)
3. Eat three nutritious meals per day
4. Exercise a minimum of 20 to 40 minutes per day. Exercise as simple as a 20-minute walk can also make you feel better. Having a favorite exercise can do more for your health than almost anything. A walk, a bike ride, stretching, hiking, surfing, kayaking... Exercise balances hormones, and we are made to move!

A good way to get ready for a change in season is to take echinacea. Echinacea is a bitter herb that strengthens your immune system. It also fills the cannabinoid receptors in the brain to make you feel better. Mediherb is my favorite brand to count on because they are the leaders in exact herbology with scientific testing to prove it.

Have you ever noticed how much a paper cut hurts? We tend to take our skin for granted until we have a paper cut or a wound. When a cut on our skin hits a nerve, that pain registers in our brain, and we say "ouch!" The same could happen if we have a burn. Nerves in our skin are important to save our lives because our skin tells us if it is too hot or cold or if something hurts.

You've heard it said that "I felt the hair on the back of my neck go up" or that "something gave me the chills." Those are all examples of how we feel our skin in different situations.

I have heard it said that 90 percent of our sympathetic nerves end in our skin. That makes sense to me because we feel everything with our skin. If our skin is numb, it indicates there is a nerve problem somewhere.

Skin is one of our vital organs. It is vital because without it, we cannot live. Just like an internal organ, our skin is part of our nervous system. If something happens to our skin, our body immediately has a warning system in place.

*Per our client:*

*"Natural Healing Center is a wonderful environment, and Shannon is a great doctor. She will meet your every need and heal you with food and natural supplements and teas. I've never had this much energy; I'm so much healthier, I've lost weight, all 100 percent naturally. Go see Shannon!!"* –Claire A.

THE 5 STRESSORS 57

> **Do your personal products such as cosmetics, shampoos, lotions, deodorants, perfumes, etc. contain harmful chemicals?**
>
> **How about your home cleaning products?**
>
> **Check out the safety of your products. Visit Enviromental Working Group**
>
> **www.EWG.org**

# PAINKILLERS: THE OPIOID EPIDEMIC

### Ephesians 2:8 AMP

*"For it is by grace [God's remarkable compassion and favor drawing you to Christ] that you have been saved [actually delivered from judgment and given eternal life]* **through faith***. And this [salvation] is not of yourselves [not through your own effort], but it is the [undeserved, gracious] gift of God." [emphasis mine]*

## Did you know?

- 60 percent of Americans (two out of five American Adults) start the day with a hot shower, a cup of coffee, and a handful of pills (four on average).
- Between 26.4 and 36 million people abuse opioids worldwide.
- An estimated 2.1 million people in the U.S. suffered from substance use disorders related to prescription opioid pain relievers in 2012.
- An estimated 467,000 people are addicted to heroin.[7]

---

7. WHO, "Dioxins and their Effect on Human Health," http://www.who.int/mediacentre/factsheets/fs225/en/. Retrieved February 25, 2018.

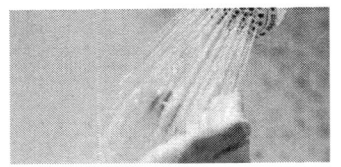

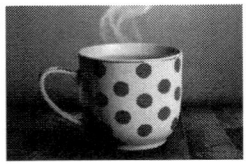

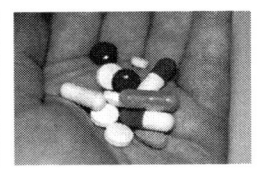

On March 29, 2017, President Donald J. Trump signed an Executive Order establishing the President's Commission on Combating Drug Addiction and the Opioid Crisis. The commission will be chaired by Governor Chris Christie and will study ways to combat and treat the scourge of drug abuse, addiction, and the opioid crisis, which was responsible for more than 50,000 deaths in 2015 and has caused families and communities across America to endure significant pain and suffering.

A common list of popular addictive opioid painkillers include:

| | |
|---|---|
| Morphine | Hydromorphone |
| Heroin | Tramadol |
| Codeine | Opium |
| Oxycodone | Fentanyl |
| Hydrocodone | Carfentanil |
| Methadone | Buprenorphine |
| | Merepidine |

Opioid painkillers mask the problem by killing the pain. They do not heal the pain in any way. Pain is a wake-up call to deal with the underlying problem. Opioid painkillers can ruin the function of your body. There is a side effect to every synthetic painkiller. There are receptors in your brain that house essential fatty acids and hormones. These opioids sit in those receptors that were meant for the fatty acids. This is likened to a party where the opioids have crashed the party and are not welcome nor useful for the brain.

Without the essential fatty acids, the nervous system suffers, and it can make your nerves raw, causing various types of pain in addition to depression and anxiety.

If you are keeping with the analogy of your body being a symphony, an opioid painkiller is like getting the symphony conductor drunk on stage while he or she is conducting the orchestra. It impairs his or her ability to conduct effectively.

The body is made to work with precision. Opioid painkillers are too strong for most situations and overpower the brain receptors. There are too many side effects from opioids. They are meant to only kill pain, but they can cause very serious, debilitating, long-lasting side effects.

Taking opioid painkillers and not addressing the cause of the pain is like a timebomb. Natural painkillers are non-addictive and can be better for you. Natural painkillers work well with the entire body. When used in conjunction with natural anti-inflammatories and natural whole food nutrition, they provide the body with complete healing.

Oftentimes, people wait too long to address their pain. It is possible to address pain before the body can no longer function. Natural healing can restore the body's function. Taking painkillers can prevent healing by masking the problem and allowing a person to function in a body that needs repairing.

Below is a chart showing the average cost of certain surgeries in Orange County, California, in 2014.

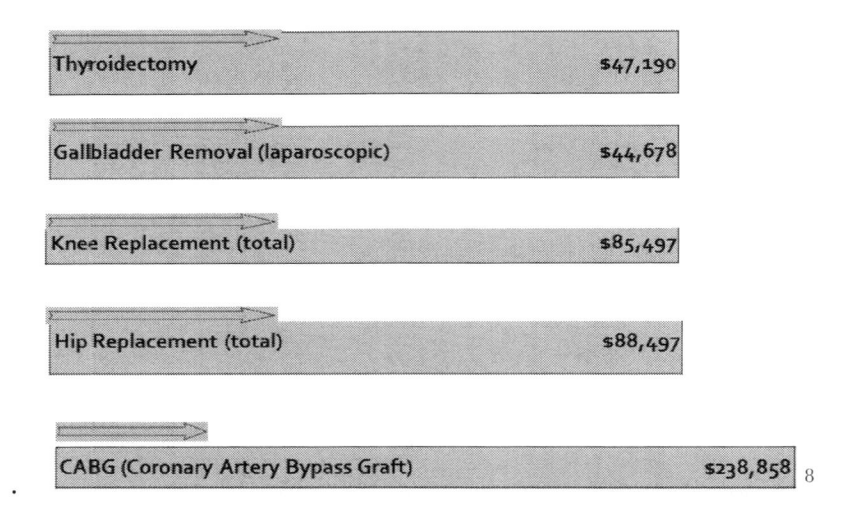

| Surgery | Cost |
|---|---|
| Thyroidectomy | $47,190 |
| Gallbladder Removal (laparoscopic) | $44,678 |
| Knee Replacement (total) | $85,497 |
| Hip Replacement (total) | $88,497 |
| CABG (Coronary Artery Bypass Graft) | $238,858 |

[8]

Health costs are the number one cause of bankruptcy in America. Understanding how to rebuild your body can help reduce your health costs. For example, some surgeries may be avoided with the proper prevention. By addressing

---

8. Health Care Atlas, OHSPD, 2014. "Common Surgery Charges at Hospitals." Orange County, CA, http://gis.oshpd.ca.gov/atlas/topics/financial/common_surgery. Retrieved February 20, 2018

inflammation immediately and getting proper whole food nutrition, in many cases, the body has the ability to heal and rebuild itself.

**Do you use antacids?**

**Click here for an example of natural healing over traditional medication.**

**http://bit.ly/2NUZUI5**

**The Choice is Yours!**

*What Our Clients Say:*

"Dr. Shannon and her staff are wonderful. She is a warm, knowledgeable practitioner who has assisted me with fatigue, weight gain, and overall joint pain. The results of her directive care began just a week into my new regimen. While the commitment has not always been easy, it has been the right decision and well worth the sacrifice of sugar, cow dairy, and grains that had me so inflamed that I hobbled to the Tylenol bottle each morning. I'm now Tylenol-free, have lost 10 pounds, and have at least 50 percent more energy. I'm an RN who works within the parameters of Western medicine, so I needed to see results of this new way of thinking. I now sing her praises daily and have begun to study her philosophies more in depth. I gave a gift certificate to my daughter for Christmas and look forward to eventually having my whole family see Dr. Shannon. If you are reading this review, I wish you great success on your endeavors. Just go for it. You will not be sorry." –Lori H.

"I broke my arm/shoulder in three places a year ago November. It was healing slowly, and I was gradually getting mobility back, and then about in October of this year, it just started to ache and hurt to exercise, so mobility took a standstill… At the suggestion of Dr. Shannon Eggleston to quit eating corn, any products with corn powder, cornstarch (Cheerios), and my favorite tortilla chips and salsa (sometimes for dinner since I thought they were pretty healthy/gluten free). Within 10 days, the pain literary disappeared and my mobility increased… I'm still off all corn. It's like a miracle. Thanks, Shannon" –Joyce B.

# PAIN IS YOUR FRIEND

**Proverbs 8:35 NLT**
*"For whoever finds me finds life and receives favor from the LORD."*

Painkillers are a bandaid. Pain is *not* the problem-pain is the symptom! Pain is a symptom of a problem. At Natural Healing Center, we investigate the reason for your pain and proceed forward to determine the cause.

We feel pain because we have nerves. From a cat scratch to a crushed neck to poor digestion or a throbbing headache, your body calls out for help.

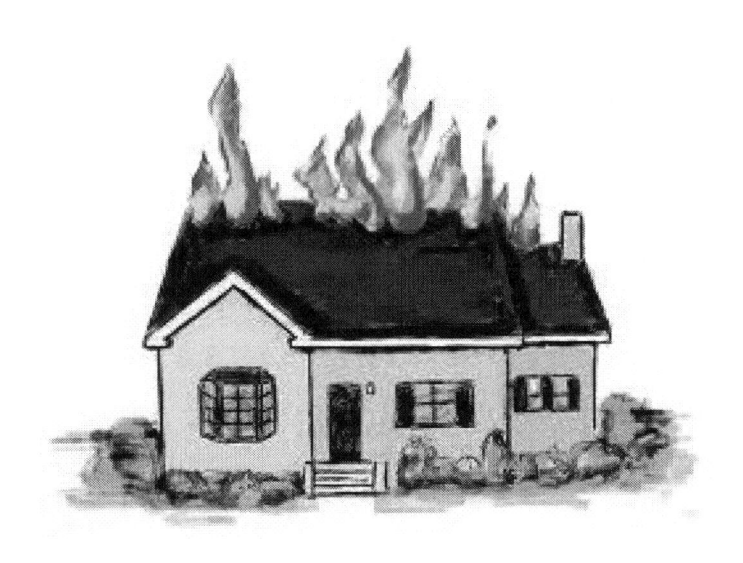

As an analogy, taking a painkiller is similar to waking up to a screaming smoke alarm as your house is in flames. Rather than extinguishing the fire, you take the batteries out of the smoke alarm and return to sleep.

Pain can be caused by many things. A stomach ache can be caused by lack of food, a concussion, a scar, dehydration, and/or foods your body doesn't like anymore. When your bones are not in alignment, it can cause a lot of pain.

Stubbing a toe can cause a limp, which puts stress on your leg and lower back that can make your neck hurt. Taking a painkiller is not as effective as soaking the stubbed toe in epsom salt water and doing proper wound care. Some people have taken painkillers so they can't feel their toe pain. They then put on their shoes and go walking and injure the toe further because they can't feel the pain.

Another example is having eye pain caused by an allergy to foods. The constant swelling and pressure deteriorates the eyes. Once the swelling is down, the eyes can heal. Taking a painkiller for the eye pain does not repair the eye; it only masks the problem.

Scars can cause pain, but taking a painkiller won't heal the scar! It needs to be massaged with the correct oil. The area of the scar needs to be stretched twice daily for 45 seconds without pain. If the scar is on a joint, gently bend it. If it is on a flat surface such as the forearm, flex it slightly. If this doesn't take care of the pain, additional methods of scar tissue therapy may be needed. Please see the chapter "The

Truth About Scars."

Pain is not easy to deal with, but pain can keep you from hurting yourself further. If you take painkillers that mask the pain so well that you don't feel any pain, you might feel a lot better, but you run the risk of further injury. Pain tells you when to stop. If you use your pain as a thermometer, you can pace yourself back to healing.

As an athlete, when you are first learning your sport, you also learn your pain level and how to avoid it by stretching out effectively without pain, drinking clean water, getting restorative sleep for eight hours a night, eating good, fresh food to rebuild your muscles, and doing your sport with joy and consistency.

When you're building strength and endurance by pushing your limits, pain tells you when you've gone too far. Pain is a tool, a coach, and a great warning system. Each individual is different. A good athlete knows his or her own pain scale. They know their own bodies, and if they've gone too far, they stop, kick it back a notch, and continue on. This may mean quitting for the day and getting a good meal and a good night's sleep or taking time off until the body heals completely, which may be three days or six weeks depending on if you have pushed yourself into an injury. Cross training can be a great way to avoid injury. Impact sports complement swimming and stretching.

Natural pain relief works with your body without any bad side effects. There are different types and levels of pain which require different solutions:

**Medi-Herb**

When pain is from a histamine reaction such as swelling and inflammation, we find out what caused the inflammation to know what remedy the body wants. If it is a food reaction, we use a food- or herb-based antihistamine. If the pain is due to injury, we use MediHerb Boswellia to take the swelling down along with MediHerb's Saligesic compound to reduce internal pain.

I use MediHerb exclusively, as their products are clinically potent and made to work. They are prepared by one of the world's premiere herbalists, Dr. Kerry Bone.

**Asea Redox**

For topical pain relief, the best remedy that we've found to date is a liquid called ASEA Redox. It goes through the skin and activates the nerve endings. It works well on everything that hurts, though it is not sold as a pain reliever. Oftentimes, when there is pain, there is nerve damage. This product works great because it activates the ends of the nerves, called telomeres. The way ASEA Redox works is by using signaling molecules. These molecules work as cellular messengers that renew your cells. ASEA can be used for topical pain, and many people drink it as well.

**Therapeutic Massage**

Therapeutic massage can also provide great pain relief.

Therapeutic massage increases circulation and oxygen to the pain site. Oxygen kills pain. There are two thoughts about clinical massage and how much pressure should be used for pain relief. One thought is to go as deep as possible no matter how much it hurts because some people think it is good for them and they like it. Each person is responsible for the pressure that they receive. The second thought is to apply medium, painless pressure to keep the swelling down and increase circulation.

When anything causes the body pain, your body will swell in that area. If you experience swelling for too long, it could prevent you from healing. By using massage with gentle pressure around the area of pain and then using medium to deep pressure on the rest of the body, it will take the swelling down. If the pain is too intense to handle any type of massage, there is a form of healing that can be performed by a professional laying their hands on you with light pressure. It was clinically proven effective in a military hospital in America. People who underwent this treatment had healed faster.

**Reflexology**

Reflexology is a science of massage that works mainly on reflex points in the hands and feet, bringing pain relief and healing to the whole body. Chinese auricular therapy uses the reflexes in the ears to bring pain relief and healing to the body. Epsom salt baths can alleviate up to 100 percent of pain. Use one pint of Epsom salt to every 50 gallons of water in a regular size bathtub for at least 20 minutes. My family uses Epsom salt to soak our hands or feet that are sore or injured to increase healing naturally. Epsom salt soaks out pain. It is important to relax and breathe while taking a bath.

**Acupressure and Acupuncture**

Acupressure and acupuncture are both Traditional Chinese Medicine methods of healing and pain relief that work by applying pressure to points along the body.

Pain is a warning system that says it's time to stop, change directions, and do something differently. I'm speaking about regular physical pain right now. Regular everyday body pains are usually nerve referred pain. A nerve being pinched in the spine will refer pain out to the body.

For example, if your neck is in pain, it may be as a result of the spine being out of alignment due to inflammation from bad foods, and/or it could be the result of overdeveloped pectoralis muscles pulling the shoulders forward.

The way the body works is like a symphony. Each individual part must do its job, keep time with the music, and play effectively. As an example, if the gall bladder is full of bad bile, there will be pain behind the shoulder blades and knees. If your feet are not kept strong, your knees and hips will not work correctly. This may cause your adrenals to release adrenaline, stopping the production of stomach acid.

If you overstretch a muscle, it will shorten, causing pain. A shortened muscle will pull the muscles it is connected to toward it. This then shortens the next muscle in line, which can then cause your entire body to stand incorrectly, ruining your posture. By stretching effectively without pain, you can re-educate the muscles to lengthen and support the body to stand correctly without being pulled one way or the other.

With the beauty of learning about Nutrition Response Testing®, a science that allows us to read the body like a book, it is possible to find the body's priority in healing.

---

**BONUS**

**Attend one of our FREE educational workshops**

**For topic and dates, visit:**

**http://naturalhealingcenter.us/events**

*Client Successes*

"I had had rheumatoid arthritis for about a year and sought medical help and tried all types of gimmicks to no avail. I was in constant pain all the time. I couldn't function or walk normally. Getting out of bed in the morning was the hardest thing for me because of the excruciating pain and depression. My life was miserable. A friend suggested Natural Healing Center (NHC), but I was hesitant due to the commitment involved. Finally, I told myself that NHC was my last resort. I had to give it a try.

On March 31, 2016, I came to Dr. Eggleston out of desperation, and I was willing to do whatever it took. Fast forward to July 29, 2017. I am now functional, walking normally, and happy. There were some surprises along the way. My skin got better. I used to use a darker foundation; now I am a shade or two lighter. I've lost weight, which I didn't expect. Actually, I am back to my pre-marital weight (22 years ago), which I never dreamed of. I am happier, less stressed, and content about my life despite the trauma I've been through.

"Before coming to Natural Healing Center, I hated getting up in the mornings because of all the pain I faced—severe, constant pain. I would sweat like a faucet out of the blue. The bottom of my feet hurt just to walk. I took pain medication three times a day, and I iced my back two to three times a day. I was very depressed. In 16 years, I never gave up because I knew there was someone on this planet who could help me. After coming to see Shannon and doing nutrition at Natural Healing Center, I have had noticeable improvement, and I look forward to starting my day with 50 percent less pain. Thanks to the Cellorgane Adrenal product, I have lost 55 pounds, and my energy level has improved. I am now more active, and my attitude has improved. Best of all, I no longer sweat like a faucet. I want to *continue improving my health for the rest of my life."* —Claudia S.

*Dr. Eggleston has helped me so much through nutrition, lifestyle changes, and coaching. I am so grateful to her for helping me to get my life back. It's been a tough journey, but it's been 100 percent worth it. Looking back, I am so glad I made the decision to come to Natural Healing Center. I'll never go back to the way I used to eat and live. Thanks to Shannon's team, I am a new, healthy woman now."* — Nancy T.

# BRAIN HEALTH

**Proverbs 2:6**
*"For the Lord gives wisdom; from his mouth come knowledge and understanding."*

The brain is where all the thinking happens. Habits are made and thoughts are captured. Our brain houses our imagination, olfactory nerves, and optic nerves so we have the ability to walk, talk, and smile. It oversees every function of the body.

Most people just think their brain is a place to hang their hat. We don't give the brain any thought until we have a brain injury or we find ourselves unable to walk or talk. The brain is connected to every action of the body. For the brain to be strong, we need to have sufficient water, essential fatty acids, and good nutrition. To keep it strong, we need good exercise and good sleep. Our whole body, including the brain, needs a day off. Taking a day of rest refreshes the brain, as it is complex and needs to unwind. Without a day off, the brain can become fragmented. Exhaustion can cause both short- and long-term memory loss, not to mention that it can ruin your mood and decision-making abilities.

To operate, the brain needs EPA and DHA, which are both essential fatty acids. Essential fatty acids are required for proper regulation of all your body systems. Having enough EPA and DHA can improve mood, memory, and focus as well as improving immune function. Sufficient EPA and DHA can also help with aging and reduce depression and the risk of dementia, Alzheimer's, and stroke. EPA and DHA can reduce the risk of coronary events by 53 percent as well as sudden death from heart attack by 90 percent. The National Institute of Health's daily recommendation of EPA and DHA is 650 mg. EPA and DHA can be found in fish oil. Standard Process provides great choices of pure, raw, organic fish oil. The most calming fish oil is the Tuna Omega-3 because it has a high DHA ratio to EPA: 240:50.

Dr. Joseph Teff, DC specializes in Chiropractic in the Middleton, WI area and has over 39 years of experience in the field of medicine. He states that your body can break down flax seed into omega-6 as well. Another form of good fats is chia seeds. Chia seeds provide a balanced combination of omegas 3, 6, and 9. There are a lot of bad fats in the American diet. Hydrogenated, hydrolyzed, and rancid fats do not work for your brain nor your body. Hydrogenated fats are fats that have had the hydrogen atom split, such as margarine. Your body does not recognize this as food. An interesting experiment you may want to try: leave a dish of margarine outside 10 yards away from a dish of butter. The insects, birds, and other animals will eat the butter but not touch the margarine because they recognize real food.

By eating enough good fats, we can ensure hormonal balance with enough exercise and oxygen. Good fats are raw. Examples include raw nuts, seeds, and olive oil. Good fats help your body remain calm. They help make up the myelin sheath that covers the nerves, and they keep your mucous membranes from drying out.

Below is a chart of the anatomy and functional areas of the brain. The brain is very complex, detailed, and exact. Each color in the brain represents a different area of function. With accurate muscle testing, such as Nutrition Response Testing®, it is possible to read the brain's needs. We can test and decipher the proper nutrition for each part of the brain, allowing the body to heal itself.

**Anatomy and Functional Areas of the Brain**

*Functional Areas of the Cerebral Cortex*

1. Visual Area: Sight, Image recognition, Image perception
2. Association Area: Short-term memory, Equilibrium, Emotion
3. Motor Function Area: Initiation of voluntary muscles
4. Broca's Area: Muscles of speech
5. Auditory Area: Hearing
6. Emotional Area: Pain, Hunger, "Fight or flight" response
7. Sensory Association Area
8. Olfactory Area: Smelling
9. Sensory Area: Sensation from muscles and skin
10. Somatosensory Association Area: Evaluation of weight, texture, temperature, etc. for object recognition
11. Wernicke's Area: Written and spoken language comprehension
12. Motor Function Area: Eye movement and orientation
13. Higher Mental Functions: Concentration, Planning, Judgment, Emotional expression, Creativity, Inhibition

*Functional Areas of the Cerebellum*

14. Motor Functions: Coordination of movement, Balance and equilibrium, Posture

---

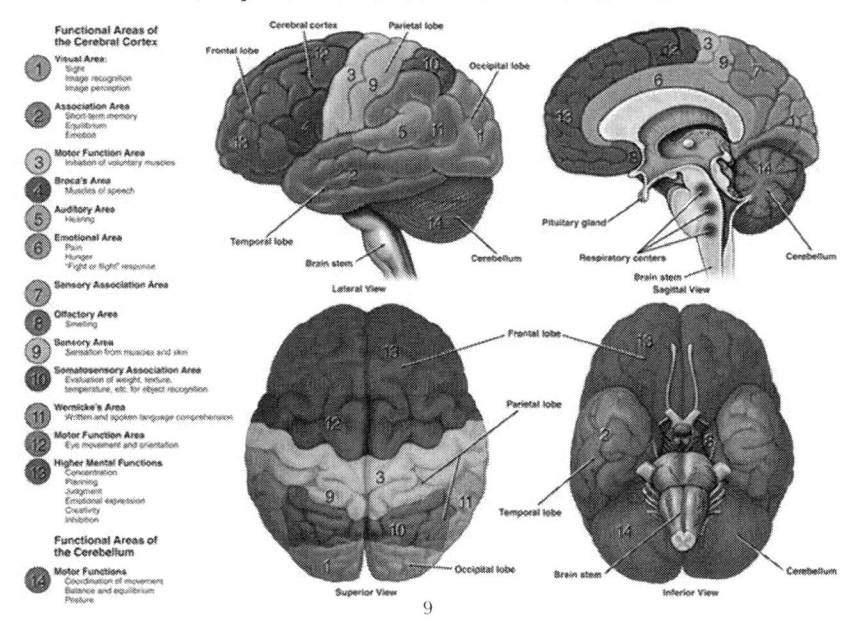

9. https://ebsco.smartimagebase.com/anatomy-and-functional-areas-of-the-brain/view-item?ItemID=1868. Retrieved March 1, 2018.

Specific fatty acids are critical to a healthy nervous system. They reduce inflammation, repair nerve cells, and improve mood, memory, and focus. They also reduce nerve and joint pain.

Optimal health focuses on improving cellular health and the function of the nervous system. Your brain's connections can become stronger or weaker over time due to many small and often repetitive physical, nutritional, or emotional events. When your brain's connections become stronger, your cognitive performance improves. Likewise, when you experience stress or nervous system interference, your cognitive performance is reduced.[10]

Maintain a lifetime of brain health. Dietary, health, genetic, metabolic, and lifestyle factors influence the structural and functional health of your brain over time. When your brain works right, your body works right.

---

10. https://www.brainspan.com/. Retrieved February 21, 2018.

## HOW IS YOUR BRAIN'S HEALTH?

### NeuroHealth Assessment Test in 4 Easy Steps:

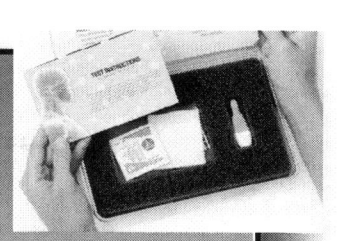

This assessment measures the capacity and efficiency of the nerve connections associated with the basic cognitive functions. How well your brain performs these functions can be an indicator of how well it is regulating your body's systems.

1. Call us to schedule an appointment to complete your assessment in our offices OR have the Assessment Kit mailed directly to you.

2. Cell Nutritional Health – Complete and send in the home blood spot test provided in the kit. This will measure your four fatty acid biomarkers.

3. Functional Brain Health – Complete this 15-minute interactive online test for measurement of attention, memory, processing speed, and cognitive flexibility.

4. Natural Healing Center will contact you directly to schedule an appointment to review your results and provide a protocol to support your goals.

Call (877) 953-3869 or visit
https://naturalhealingcenter.us/contact

*What Our Clients Say:*

"I recently found out about the Natural Healing Center while I was looking for a holistic approach to my inflammation issues. When I met Shannon Eggleston and she applied the Nutrition Response Technique on me, I didn't quite understand. But after a few weeks, I could feel the difference by following her instructions and taking the whole food supplements she advised me to take. I feel much better now! I definitely recommend a visit with her." –Regina C.

"After seeing Dr. Shannon for a couple of months, I can tell you that I have never felt better in my life. I was not feeling the best when I started seeing her, and it was really affecting my mood. Well, after just a few weeks of treatment, I noticed a lift in my mood and attitude. I began to feel great, joyful, and overall just really happy again. Who knew that I could feel this great? I have tons of energy, and I sleep for a full eight hours with no problem. And as a bonus, my weight continues to balance itself effortlessly.

I also recommend Dr. Shannon to my clients since she really is the best, and you can tell she and her staff have one mission in life: to help as many people as possible get healthy and live their best lives ever. Going to her office is a joyful experience as well. I really dislike going to Western doctors' offices; the environment feels sterile and like going there is not really helping much. The difference at Natural Healing Center is the high vibration of the office, and one can feel real healing is going on in that place. Anyway, I just can't say enough great things about Dr. Shannon and Natural Healing Center." –Nayelli C.

# MENTAL HEALTH

**Proverbs 1:5 KJV**
*"A wise man will hear and increase in learning, And a man of understanding will acquire wise counsel."*

Mental illness is nothing to be ashamed of. It is a medical problem just like heart disease or diabetes. With over 26 years in business helping people feel better by using food as medicine, the one thing that always surprises me is how much happier people are after only three weeks of eating whole foods, drinking clean water, and rubbing their scars.

I have seen very depressed people become well this way. I have also witnessed people with high anxiety become well. Eating green vegetables, good sources of protein, seeds, and nuts can provide most of the nutrients that you need to be well. Being well means functioning optimally and happily.

Nutritional deficiencies cause depression, nausea, mood swings, sleep deficiencies, and illness.

Processed sugar can cause inflammation and tissue damage in the body and brain. The average American eats 150 pounds of processed sugar a year. Sugar feeds bacteria. Sugar feeds cancer. Sugar feeds candida, causing swelling and inflammation. Candida, also known as a yeast infection, feeds on sugar in the gut and causes leaky gut. With leaky gut, the bacteria from the intestines leaks into the bloodstream and causes autoimmune responses and allergies. Allergies cause inflammation, resulting in a swollen brain. A swollen brain results in brain fog and lack of oxygen. Lack of oxygen causes deterioration and disease. To reverse deterioration and disease, we encourage an anti-inflammatory diet, a balanced regime of rest and gentle exercise, and a positive mindset.

An anti-inflammatory diet is void of grains and sugars of any kind. Absolutely no processed foods such as soda, juices, cookies, cakes, candies, or ice cream. No caffeine or dairy products. Imagine living on a farm a long time ago where you ate only what you grew. Bacon and eggs for breakfast, salad for lunch, and steak and sweet potatoes with vegetables for dinner. This is the beginning of an anti-inflammatory diet.

The book *Gut and Psychology Syndrome* by Dr. Natasha Campbell-McBride explains natural treatments for autism, dyslexia, ADHD, depression, and schizophrenia. This book is a wonderful example of how good nutrition can help heal the body and mind.

*"All disease begins in the gut."* –Hippocrates, 460–370 BC

The experts at Harvard Medical School talk about how a healthy gut leads to a healthy brain. The cells in the gut mimic the cells in the brain. Serotonin is a neurotransmitter that helps regulate sleep and appetite, mediate moods, and inhibit pain. Since about 95 percent of your serotonin is produced in your gastrointestinal tract, and your gastrointestinal tract is lined with a hundred million nerve cells, or neurons, it makes sense that the inner workings of your digestive system don't just help you digest food but also guide your emotions.

What's more, the function of these neurons—and the production of neurotransmitters like serotonin—is highly influenced by the billions of "good" bacteria that make up your intestinal microbiome. These bacteria play an essential role in your health. They protect the lining of your intestines and ensure they provide a strong barrier against toxins and "bad" bacteria. They limit inflammation, improve how well you absorb nutrients from your food, and activate neural pathways that travel directly between the gut and the brain.[11]

Stop the madness. If you are told you have a chemical imbalance and the most important thing you can do for yourself is to take your medication for life, you should first consider how to reverse the cause of your imbalance. Dietary change is a powerful—if not the most powerful—means of effecting the microbiome and gut-brain signaling.

By taking probiotic supplements, eating sauerkraut, or drinking low-sugar kombucha, you can rebuild the intestinal flora, creating good bacteria. By having good bacteria outnumber the bad bacteria, the intestinal tract is clean and healthy.

---

11. Eva Selhub, MD, "Nutritional Psychiatry: Your Brain on Food," https://www.health.harvard.edu/blog/nutritional-psychiatry-your-brain-on-food-201511168626. Retrieved March 5, 2018.

Many people think that mental health depends on treating just the brain. The body is a whole; there are no separate parts. Eating an anti-inflammatory diet to keep inflammation down is not only good for the body, but it is good for the brain as well.

Psych meds can have serious side effects such as depression and suicide and can be habit-forming. Common side effects include:

- Drowsiness
- Dizziness
- Restlessness
- Weight gain (the risk is higher with some atypical antipsychotic medicines)
- Dry mouth
- Constipation
- Nausea
- Vomiting

Selective serotonin reuptake inhibitors, also known as SSRIs, are some of the most widely prescribed psychotropic drugs. They include citalopram (Celexa), escitalopram oxalate (Lexapro), fluoxetine (Prozac), fluvoxamine (Luvox), paroxetine HRI (Paxil), and sertraline (Zoloft).

On a daily basis, we are exposed to harmful toxins that affect the performance of our brain and body. An example of some toxins we are exposed to daily are pesticides, bleach, cleaning fluid, acetone, diesel, chlorine and fluoride. These are also known as endocrine disruptors, as they may interfere with the production or activity of hormones in the endocrine system. Avoid exposure to these toxins at all costs. Eat organically, choose personal products without chemicals, and choose natural cleaning products such as tea tree oil, vinegar, toothpaste without fluoride, water filters, etc. The Environmental Working Group at https://www.ewg.org is a powerful guide to help you discover products that you can use to replace harmful ones.

The brain needs minerals and fats to function properly. By going off sugar and inflammatory foods completely and getting your circulation going by rubbing your scars, your body and brain can heal.

# NUTRITION RESPONSE TESTING®

**Proverbs 8:33 NIV**
*"Listen to my instruction and be wise; do not disregard it."*

**What Is Nutrition Response Testing®?**

Nutrition Response Testing® is a non-invasive way of analyzing the body through muscle testing to determine underlying nutritional causes of interference and stress that can affect a person's health.

It obtains critical information about bodily function from the autonomic nervous system (ANS). Autonomic refers to something that occurs involuntarily. Bodily functions like eye blinking, heart and breathing rates, digestive metabolism, immune response, hormone regulation, and so forth are regulated by the ANS. There are two controls to the ANS:

1. Sympathetic
2. Parasympathetic

Think of them as your body's accelerator (sympathetic control) and brake (parasympathetic control): our "go" pedal and "whoa" pedal. When our bodies are healthy and in balance, these systems function properly and are in tune with

> **How Do Your Supplements Stack Up?**
>
> **Find out the difference between natural, raw, organic whole food supplements and synthetic vitamins.**
>
> **How to Read Labels:**
> http://bit.ly/2LuVW7i
>
> **The Lure of Synthetic Vitamins:**
> http://bit.ly/2zJq1yG
>
> **Proof Positive for Throwing Away:**
> http://bit.ly/2LjVfko

one another; the sympathetic dominates when we are active, the parasympathetic when we are resting.

These regulators are responsible for healthy functioning, including our ability to heal. It is when there is an imbalance, blockage, or interference that we experience symptoms such as allergies, acid reflux, high blood pressure, chronic pain, headaches, and the like. Think of these symptoms as check engine lights or alarm bells. These balances can be corrected safely, naturally, and effectively by accessing the ANS.[12]

This approach to healing balances the body through diet, whole food supplements, and homeopathy to help support the body and the immune system. In turn, your body is set free from the stressors that interfere with normal functioning and is finally able to heal and repair itself properly.

Nutrition Response Testing® uses neurological reflexes and acupuncture points selected from the ancient Chinese system of acupuncture. These reflexes are the body's way of showing what areas are not functioning optimally and could use more support.

Nutrition Response Testing® analysis is performed by applying pressure to your extended arm with one hand and pressure to a specific reflex area on the body with the other

---

12. Rosen, Paul J. *The Great Health Heist*, Cornelius, NC, Warren Publishing Inc., 2007. 68–69.

"Nutrition Response Testing®" is a Registered Service Mark owned by Dr. Freddie Ulan and is used with his permission.

hand. If the tested reflex is stressed, the nervous system will respond by reducing energy to the extended arm, causing the arm to weaken. This weakness indicates underlying stress in that area that may be affecting health and well-being. To help the body respond to this stress, Designed Clinical Nutrition can be applied.

## What Is Designed Clinical Nutrition?

Specific nutritional supplement formulas are tested against those weakened areas to find which ones bring your reflexes back to strength and balance. This way, a unique program is tailor-made for you and created based on the responses that your body gives during the analysis.

Designed Clinical Nutrition is concentrated raw, organic, whole food in a tablet, capsule, or tea prepared using a process that preserves all of the active enzymes and vital components that make the body work as nature intended. These real food supplements have been designed to specifically match the needs of the body. Designed Clinical Nutrition does not consist of over-the-counter vitamins. Over-the-counter vitamins are pharmaceutically produced in a laboratory and are not derived from whole foods, often causing you to be even more deficient and nutritionally out-of-balance, which may even lead to health problems. Once you begin to follow the recommended program, you could see results in as little as four to six weeks.

*What Our Clients Say:*

*"Shannon has worked with me to greatly improve my health. Her approach is paying off. I told Shannon I wanted to have improved vision and also get rid of my dry eyes so I could maybe wear contacts again. This week, I went to my opthamologist, and he told me my prescription needed to change because my eyes had improved so much he needed to give me a weaker prescription. Also, my eyes are moist again, and I can wear contacts. Shannon really understands how to treat her clients' medical issues. You cannot go wrong if you see her."* –Kim P.

Many of our health problems are the result of years and years of doing the wrong things for our bodies. Therefore, it is important to keep in mind that some cases take a bit longer to resolve than others. Your body will prioritize and gradually reveal all the issues that need to be addressed. One by one, as you eliminate toxic foods from your diet, shed toxins from your system, and restore your cells with healthy foods and supplements, your organs and systems will grow cleaner, stronger, and more stable, and your health will be restored. Generally, one month of healing is needed per year of disease.

*What Our Clients Say:*

*"After seeking help from countless health practitioners and never getting any better, I was referred to the Natural Healing Center by a friend. Tired of feeling so awful all the time, nowhere near a path to feeling better nor knowing what the root of the cause was for my failing health, I decided to give it a try. I thank God I was led to such an amazing person with such insight into how the body works. She was able to finally*

*determine what was going on and why I had so many different issues going on. It's unfortunate it took this long to find someone who could get to the root of the problem but, thankfully, we did. I now feel like I have my health back. No more lethargy, pain, digestion issues, brain fog, adrenal issues, food allergies, or weight issues. If you're tired of not feeling well, you should seriously consider The Natural Healing Center."*
—Amanda R.

# BLOCKS AND SWITCHES

*"No cookies, cakes, candies, or ice cream."* –Dr. Bryman

What makes Nutrition Response Testing® so unique is that it checks that the nervous system is not "blocked" or "switched." If any part of the nervous system, which includes 156 different circuits, is blocked or switched, you won't respond properly to any diet or supplement changes because the body is not open to healing. If someone is blocked or switched, they can fluctuate between getting better and then worse over and over, or they simply won't respond properly at all.

Your autonomic nervous system (the part that operates without you thinking about it) has the ability to regulate the "brakes" and "gas" of your body, sending more or less energy to support the body depending upon where it is needed. When someone is running, his or her body needs to increase its energy or up-regulate. If a person is sleeping or watching TV, the body needs to down-regulate.

"Switching" is when the nervous system becomes dysregulated and is in a state of confusion. It may actually do the opposite of what one would normally expect; it "runs" when it should rest and vice versa. This switching needs to be corrected before the body can respond properly to healing programs. If it is left unaddressed, you can potentially have the opposite response to what is intended.

A body in poor health cannot adjust to changing conditions. It is stuck in some level of "rest" or "run" and has lost its ability to adapt to outside influences. This interferes with its ability to heal itself, and is, therefore, the highest priority to correct. People cannot respond to treatment without first addressing blocks and switches.

All *blocked* regulation and *switched* confusion is caused by stressors that interfere with the normal nervous system function. A stressor is anything that suppresses the immune system or nervous system function. It can be any type of immune challenge. We identify which stressor is causing the block or switch and help the body remove it with the specific supplements or remedy.

*Client Successes:*

*"I met Shannon several years ago, hoping she could help me in my health issues, and it was a success! Her approach takes all the guesswork out of finding what was wrong with my physical health. Thank you for all the great support and wisdom you share."* —Marcus Barrera, Professional Surfing Coach

*"Shannon is amazing and intuitive. I went in to see her after three separate ER visits for the same health problem. After one visit, I followed her directions and have been feeling healthier, happier, and more awake. I can't recommend her enough. Any chronic, nagging problem or annoying pain can be gotten rid of for good. All pain is gone, and I've lost weight as a result of the treatment. Can't go wrong."* —Cat C.

*"Shannon, you are a hidden gem! I am so happy and grateful to have been referred to you. I knew using the body testing methods you use to create a natural and tailored treatment plan was right up my alley. I have been frustrated for years not knowing why I (an RN and avid health and nutrition enthusiast) had a huge deficit in energy. I couldn't rationally legitimize my fatigue and overall depressed, lack-luster state of health. By traditional medical standards, I was healthy. I am so appreciative that you helped me at the pit of my despair. I couldn't eat!!! I had horrible intestinal pain and spasms. I was really at a loss and didn't know how to help myself.*

*To get to the point I am very pleased to learn about the imbalances I was unknowingly subjecting my body to. The metal from my belly ring was disrupting the energetic health of nine different organs. Unbelievable. My metal underwire bra was not helping. As a woman, the cost of my hormone balance was so not worth it. I have learned the importance of allowing the demands of the human body to circulate energy for health and balance. I honor this now and no longer take this demand for granted. For me, this was correlated to the multiple food intolerances and underactive thyroid Shannon identified. Giving my body the nutrients it was deficient in with supplements and getting rid of the metal I had been wearing for years made me feel like a million bucks. It was also absolutely necessary to avoid certain foods, as I was healing my stomach and intestines. I had forgotten what it feels like to feel vivacious and abundant in energy. I love that you showed me how to eat right for me and only me. Thank you. #Losethemetal!! –Leslie M.*

# NOW: NUTRITION, OXYGEN, AND WATER

**Proverbs 2:20 NIV**
*"Thus you will walk in the ways of the good and keep to the paths of the righteous."*

**Feel Better NOW Using the Power of Nutrition, Oxygen, and Water**

**Nutrition**

The power of NOW is amazing! Nutrition is what your body gets out of the food you eat. Better nutrition is when you eat food that is fresh and organically grown or raised without antibiotics.

When you eat peacefully and chew each bite at least 20 times, your body will absorb nutrition better. Eating slower is better than eating faster. Taking small bites and chewing thoroughly is best. Eating slowly is good for you because it causes your body to relax. When you are in a hurry, your body goes into a fight and flight response, and your stomach acid stops forming. Without stomach acid, the food cannot be processed, and nutrients cannot be absorbed.

Organic vegetables such as chard, lettuce, celery, asparagus, broccoli, etc. should comprise 50 percent to 75 percent of your plate, followed by organic protein such as chicken, beef, fish, and lamb. Complex carbs can be 25 percent of your plate and include yams, zucchini, squash, and pumpkin. Finally, good fats such as avocado, olive oil, raw nuts, chia seeds, and flax seeds are important to keep you full and satiated. They also keep you from craving sugar.

**Oxygen**

Are you in the habit of not breathing? It sounds funny, but have you ever caught yourself holding your breath? Oxygen is necessary to calm your nerves. Take a deep breath, relax, and exhale. That is supposed to be a normal function. By breathing evenly throughout the day, your body is calmer and better able to handle every situation.

Oxygen kills disease. Oxygen calms our nerves and helps us to repair everything in our body. Getting daily exercise is a great way to oxygenate the body. Whether you like to walk, bike, dance, or do a sport, exercise is a great way to increase your intake of oxygen. Exercise balances your hormones and relieves stress. Daily walking, stretching, or dancing is good for you.

## Practice Breathing for Relaxation and Pain Control

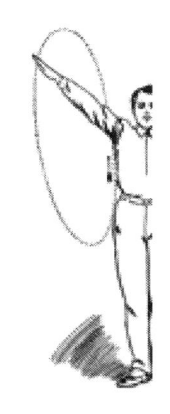

1. Arm rotation backward in your range of motion, one arm at a time

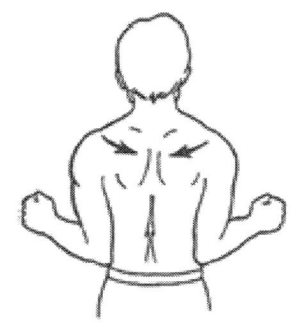

2. Shoulder pinches backward while exhaling

## Water

Drink clean, pure spring water without any additives. The body needs water to clean itself, so the cleaner your water is, the cleaner your body will be. Your body is made up of

75 percent water. If you don't have enough water, you may become dehydrated. Dehydration causes headaches, nausea, stomach aches, flu-like symptoms, and blackouts. You may also experience dry mouth, dry eyes, and dry mucous membranes.

Drink water to increase your health! The cleaner your water, the less work your body has to do. Water will energize you better than coffee. Drinking half your bodyweight in ounces of water is a good start!

**Drink Half Your Body Weight in Ounces**

## DAILY WATER INTAKE

| WEIGHT | WATER | WATER BOTTLE 16.9 OUNCES |
|---|---|---|
| 80 lbs | 40 oz. | 2 |
| 100 lbs | 50 oz. | 3 |
| 120 lbs | 60 oz. | 4 |
| 140 lbs | 70 oz. | 4 |
| 160 lbs | 80 oz. | 5 |
| 180 lbs | 90 oz. | 5 |
| 200 lbs | 100 oz. | 6 |
| 220 lbs | 110 oz. | 7 |
| 240 lbs | 120 oz. | 7 |
| 260 lbs | 130 oz. | 8 |
| 280 lbs | 140 oz. | 8 |
| 300 lbs | 150 oz. | 9 |
| 320 lbs | 160 oz. | 10 |

Drink pure spring water and filter your water to remove these common toxins:

- Fluoride

- Chlorine
- Lead
- Mercury
- Chromium-6
- Arsenic
- Pesticides
- Insecticides
- Chemicals
- And more

As discussed previously in the chapter on the five stressors, chlorine is one of the top five stressors to the body. As a halogen, chlorine is a highly efficient disinfectant and is added to public water supplies. Chlorine kills disease-causing pathogens such as bacteria, viruses, and protozoans that commonly grow in water supply reservoirs, on the walls of water mains, and in storage tanks.[13]

Yet, according to the U.S. Council on Environmental Quality, the cancer risk to people who drink chlorinated water is 93 percent higher than for those whose water does not contain chlorine.[14]

---

13. Wikipedia, "Water Chlorination," https://en.wikipedia.org/wiki/Water_chlorination. Retrieved February 28, 2018.
14. Mercola, "Water Chlorination: Is Chlorine in Drinking Water Safe?" https://www.mercola.com/downloads/bonus/chlorine/default.htm. Retrieved March 1, 2018.

Since your skin is your largest organ and highly porous, it is advisable to install a shower filter to remove chlorine in addition to the common toxins listed above.

I like the filters offered by Clearly Filtered. They are one of the few manufacturers that remove 98 percent of fluoride as well as many other major contaminants. You can visit their site at https://www.clearlyfiltered.com/ to view test reports on water filtration.

*Client Successes:*

*"I brought my husband to Dr. Shannon six years ago. His blood pressure was 200/110. He was on five cardiac medications (top dosage), and his cardiologist said, "I don't know what else to do for you." The doctor agreed to a nutritionist. After four weeks of detoxing, removing bad food, and replacing it with good food per Dr. Shannon's instructions, his blood pressure was down to 130/80. I highly recommend Dr. Shannon to anyone who is currently consuming the American diet."* –Dr. Becky E.

*"Rob Cope here to tell you my personal transformation. January 26, 2017, I was diagnosed with stage two melanoma skin cancer. My regular physician wanted $30,000 for radiation, chemo, and surgery to cut a softball size of tissue from the middle of my back. I chose a different path. I went to a holistic place called Natural Healing Center. My weight was 258.6 pounds, and my diet was a horrific acidic pH. I was drinking Diet Cokes for breakfast and eating chili dogs for lunch and greasy hamburgers for dinner with milkshakes and candy bars for treats. I did a 360° to green vegetables, 100 ounces of water per day, fish, and berries only. My latest pH was 7.8, and I now weigh 187 pounds. The skin cancer is gone. I have perfect blood pressure at 110/70, no problem with triglycerides, uric acid, or cholesterol.*

*I'm staying on this healthy path the rest of my life, as my waist went from 44 inches to 36 inches, and I sleep much better too. Nutrition, God, and Dr. Eggleston have helped complete my 360° life change, and I can't thank them enough!"* —Rob C.

---

**Are You Addicted to Sugar?**

**Take this quiz to see if you are sugar addicted.**

**Sugar Quiz:**
**http://bit.ly/2Lo5owQ**

**Why No White Sugar:**
**http://bit.ly/2LtPKfU**

# HARROWER'S CHART: HOW THE ENDOCRINE SYSTEM WORKS

**Proverbs 4:23 NIV**
*"Above all else, guard your heart,
for everything you do flows from it."*

Imagine a wagon wheel. Imagine that each spoke is a different organ in your body. The middle of the wagon wheel is the thyroid, and the wheel itself is the skin, representing the largest organ. This wagon wheel represents the way that your body's organs work together in the system called the endocrine system.

Each organ is important to every other organ in the system. Michael E. Greer, MD is an integrative medicine expert focused on holistic, herbal, homeopathic, and naturopathic solutions for health. He lectures internationally at medical conferences and seminars to educate doctors about integrative medicine. He explains that when you have sand in your eye, every single part of your body knows that you have sand in your eye. It's like your mind is saying, "There is sand in your eye! There is sand in your eye!" It is an upset to the entire system.

The same is true of any other emergency in the body. It's just that we have learned how to go into overdrive and ignore our bodies' symptoms. The body gives us warnings in small symptoms, and as the problem gets bigger, the symptoms get bigger. Meanwhile, there is a panic going on under our skin that we don't even know about because it is not as obvious as sand in our eyes.

Sometimes, symptoms such as pain—back pain, stomach pain, headaches, etc.—are very loud warning signals.

Much like a car making noises, if we are trained to listen, we will spend much less money on repairs if we take the car in right away rather than wait. We all know that cars need water, oil, and check-ups. Our bodies are the same way! We need water, oil, and check-ups too.

A trained mechanic can listen to an engine and know which part is misfiring. The same is true for a trained practitioner. Understanding the endocrine system and how it works is imperative to help the body work as a whole. Hence, the word "holistic." God made us, and His work is perfect: He knit you together in your mother's womb.

Dr. Henry R. Harrower was a pioneer of endocrinology during the early half of the 20th century. Dr. Harrower's chart is a great example of how many organs can work together to form a perfect orchestra, a perfect symphony—each organ doing its own part. As in a symphony, each instrument works together to present the whole work of art. Another great analogy for the way the body works is a watch. Every watch has a maker. Each part of the watch is almost useless without the others, but when you put them all together, the time

HARROWER'S CHART 107

peace runs perfectly.

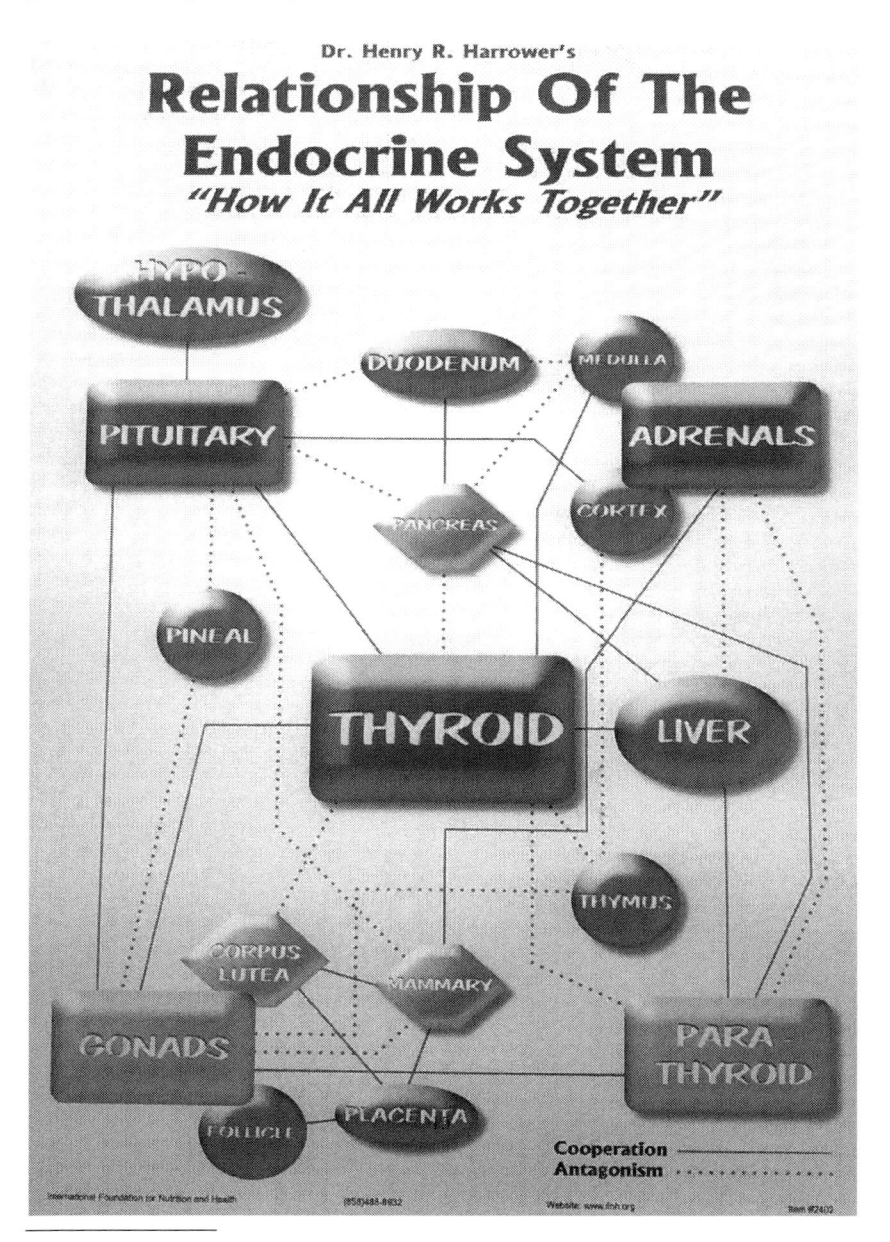

**Dr. Henry R. Harrower's**
# Relationship Of The Endocrine System
*"How It All Works Together"*

---

15. http://ifnh.org/wp-content/uploads/2015/06/Harrowers-Endocrine-Poster-pic-taken-with-phone.jpg

*A Comment from our Client:*

"*I am so blessed every time I visit Shannon! She is so knowledgeable and thorough. She was able to resolve my hair loss, low thyroid, "tennis elbow," and adrenal fatigue as well as some other issues I didn't know I had! I have much more energy now and clearer thinking than before. The improvement in my health is well worth every penny I paid. I highly recommend her!*" –Susan C.

# THE BODY AS A WHOLE: MIND, BODY, AND SOUL

**Psalms 2:10 NIV**
*"For wisdom will enter your heart,
and knowledge will be pleasant to your soul."*

110    SCARS AND ROADBLOCKS TO HEALING

16

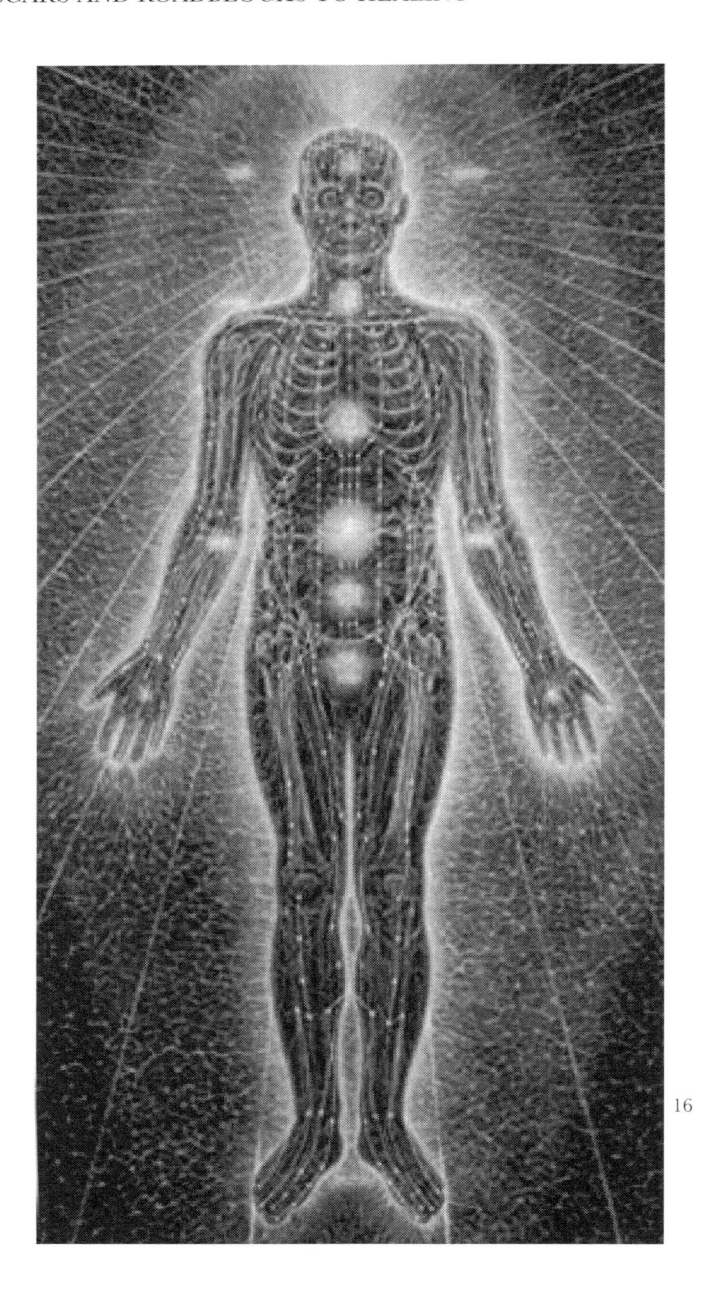

16. Richard Boyd, "The Concept of Human Energy Fields," 2015, http://energeticsinstitute.com.au/concept-of-human-energy-fields/. Retrieved January 8, 2018.

# THE BODY AS A WHOLE

We are made up of flesh, blood, bones, tissue, an emotional heart, a mind, and a soul. The body is the flesh and is made up of solid matter. The emotional heart emits feelings. The mind and soul are ethereal. The body has its own mind and inheritance, inheritance meaning genetics, preferences in sleep and food or the way you do certain things such as walking or your mannerisms.

The emotional heart is also known as the pericardium in Traditional Chinese Medicine. The pericardium is a meridian, and it is affected by how happy or unhappy your heart is.

The mind is always thinking, and not always correctly. Sometimes, it can feel like an open door to the whole universe. It is good to train the mind to decipher what is good and what is bad. It is also good to teach the mind to ignore minutia (useless information) and bad thoughts. Information comes in through the eyes, and the brain immediately starts making up stories about the information it sees. It is important to train the mind to sift through what information is pertinent and what is not. Ideally, one would train the brain to not make up stories. Oftentimes, they are lies that do not serve your best interest.

The soul is your spirit. It is the part of you that craves deep, loving connections. The soul is who you really are. It is important to have a connection with God, who loves us and feeds our souls by guarding us and guiding us to our destiny. No one knows us like God knows us. We get our bodies in a lot of trouble trying to soothe our souls while we are looking for that deep, loving relationship that only God can provide. Some people overshop to feel better, while others overmedicate, overeat, drive too fast, or sabotage themselves in seeking relief. In the Bible, King David spoke to his soul saying, "Why, my soul, are you downcast? Why so disturbed within me? Put your hope in God, for I will yet praise him, my Savior and my God." Psalms 43:5 NIV

# FAITH AND ENCOURAGEMENT

*"Now faith is the substance of things hoped for, the evidence of things not seen."* Hebrews 11:1 King James Version (KJV)

**Hebrews 11:1 NIV**

"Faith means being sure (the assurance or the tangible reality or the sure foundation) of the things we hope for and knowing that something is real even if we do not see it (the conviction/assurance/evidence about things not seen)." [emphasis mine]

**Philippians 1:6 NIV**

"He who began a good work in you will be faithful to complete it."

God made us for His friendship and company to do His good service. Each of us is born for a reason. Since time began, God has had a vision for your life. Knowing our purpose gives us strength to do the right things. Spending time alone with God strengthens our relationship with Him. We are made to be in relationship with Him and each other.

**Isaiah 43:7 KJV**

"[Even] every one that is called by my name: for I have

created him for my glory, I have formed him; yea, I have made him."

Faith goes beyond just salvation; it enables God to work both in and through us. Faith helps us grow. It can change lives, move mountains, and allow miracles to happen. Here are some Bible quotes to encourage you:

**Hebrews 11:1 NLT**

"Faith is the confidence that what we hope for will actually happen; it gives us assurance about things we cannot see."

**Matthew 17:20 ESV**

"... For truly, I say to you, if you have faith like a grain of mustard seed, you will say to this mountain, 'Move from here to there,' and it will move, and nothing will be impossible for you."

**Romans 1:16–17 KJV**

"For I am not ashamed of the gospel of Christ: for it is the power of God unto salvation to every one that believeth; to the Jew first, and also to the Greek. For therein is the righteousness of God revealed from faith to faith: as it is written, The just shall live by faith."

**Matthew 9:20–22 NLT**

"Just then a woman who had suffered for twelve years with constant bleeding came up behind Him. She touched the fringe of His robe, for she thought, 'If I can just touch His robe, I will be healed.' Jesus turned around, and when He saw her He said, 'Daughter, be encouraged! ***Your faith has made you well.***' And the woman was healed at that moment." [emphasis mine]

## II Corinthians 5:7 NKJV

"For we walk by faith, not by sight."

## James 2:14–17 NLT

"What good is it, dear brothers and sisters, if you say you have faith but don't show it by your actions? Can that kind of faith save anyone? Suppose you see a brother or sister who has no food or clothing, and you say, 'Good-bye and have a good day; stay warm and eat well'—but then you don't give that person any food or clothing. What good does that do?

"So you see, faith by itself isn't enough. Unless it produces good deeds, it is dead and useless."

## I Corinthians 16:13–14 NIV

"Be on guard; stand firm in the faith; be courageous; be strong. Do everything in love."

## Matthew 21:21–22 AMPC

"And Jesus answered them, 'Truly I say to you, if you have faith (a firm relying trust) and do not doubt, you will not only do what has been done to the fig tree, but even if you say to this mountain, 'Be taken up and cast into the sea,' it will be done. And whatever you ask for in prayer, having faith and [really] believing, you will receive."

## Ephesians 6:16 ESV

"In all circumstances take up the shield of faith, with which you can extinguish all the flaming darts of the evil one."

## I Corinthians 13:13 NLT

"Three things will last forever—faith, hope, and love—and the greatest of these is love."

## Jeremiah 29:11-13 NIV

"For I know the plans I have for you,' declares the LORD, plans to prosper you and not to harm you, plans to give you hope and a future. Then you will call on me and come and pray to me, and I will listen to you. You will seek me and find me when you seek me with all your heart."

God has healing powers. Jesus said "get up and walk" after the crippled man's friends lowered him through the roof and ceiling into a crowded room to be healed. Those friends had faith. Their faith allowed him to be healed. If it weren't for their courage to rip the roof apart, he might have never gotten the healing from Jesus. The people you surround yourself with make a difference. Make sure the people you are with are ones of faith and encouragement. They will have your back.

Have courage. The God of the Universe has plans for you to prosper even if it may not feel like it at the time. Speak life over self, family, and friends. When you don't feel well, you can say the truth: "this body heals in Jesus' name." There's healing in the name of Jesus.

Chains hold us back from healing. Sometimes, we are chained to our pasts. Sometimes, our belief systems chain us. When Jesus was walking by the cemetery, there was a man running around with shackles, out of his mind. After an encounter with Jesus, he was healed and free of his chains.

> **Let go of your past, give the things that torment you to Jesus, and rely on Him for everything.**

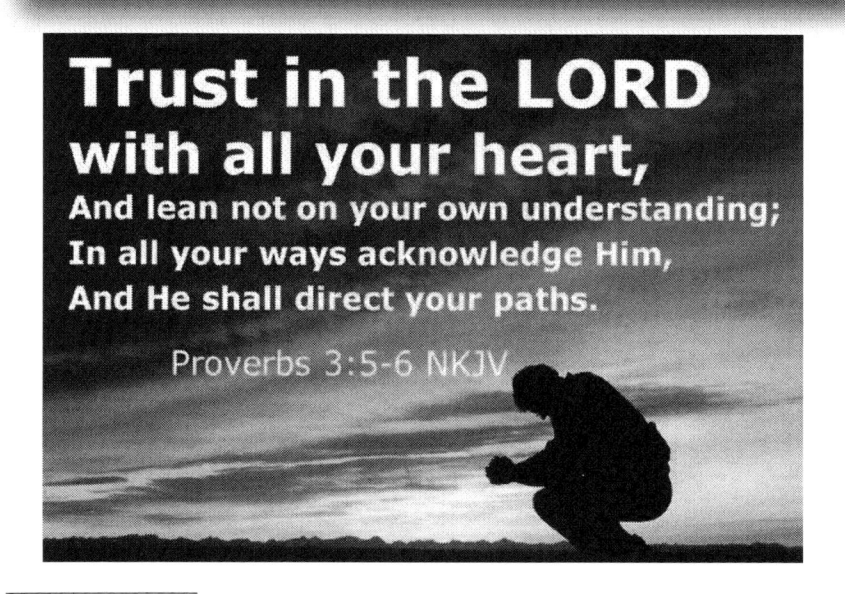

**Trust in the LORD with all your heart,
And lean not on your own understanding;
In all your ways acknowledge Him,
And He shall direct your paths.**

Proverbs 3:5-6 NKJV

---

17. http://www.tellthelordthankyou.com/blog/2017/1/11/proverbs-35-6-trust-god. Retrieved February 28, 2018.

*A Comment from our Client:*

"I am amazed at the results. My body, for the first time in my life, is in true 100 percent good health. It's free of toxins that I didn't even know were the root cause of my joint pain. I have more energy, I am making better decisions, and overall, being healthy truly makes my surroundings a lot more pleasing. My business has skyrocketed, and my kids are glad to have Mom back playing ball and surfing with them. Being in great health and filtering all the old junk from inside actually has made me a better wife, mother, boss, person, and mentor. I wish I did this ages ago! AMEN! Thank you for giving me my life back." –Emma R.

# ABOUT SHANNON EGGLESTON

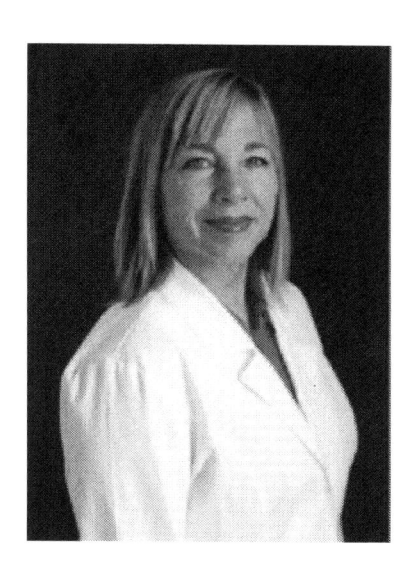

**Naturopath, Holistic Health Practitioner (HHP), #1 Best Selling Author**

Shannon is a graduate of Advanced Clinical Training in Nutrition Response Testing®. Her studies include Mueller College of Holistic Health, the Southern College of Naturopathy, and the Guang An Men Hospital in China. It was in China where she came to realize the benefits of Chinese Medicine, organic foods and supplements.

An established holistic speaker and author, Shannon is a lecturer for Standard Process on nutrition and has spoken at several corporations, schools, universities, and associations. She has volunteered for many medical mission trips working alongside medical doctors, surgeons, and nurses.

Fun fact: Shannon was raised in Hawaii and assisted Ironman Triathlon competitors with hydration measures during the race and massage therapy after the race. She also provided nutrition and muscle therapy for the physically demanding commercial salmon fishing industry. You can find her surfing most mornings and sometimes hula dancing!

# BONUS

**How to Be Jet Lag-Free**

I learned how to be jet lag-free from my acupressure teacher, Ramona Moody. She taught me how to avoid jet lag on the way to China, and it worked! I was operating on China's time zone without any problem even after a 14-hour flight.

Because the jet lag formula worked so well on the way to China, I took it for granted that I could handle the trip back without the jet lag formula. As a result, I suffered jet lag exhaustion severely for a solid two weeks!

The theory of jet lag is this: every two hours of the day, a part of your body heals. The science of the jet lag free theory is to activate the points on the body as if you are in the time zone where you are traveling to.

Once you get on the plane, you can start activating the points on the body. Rub or pat one side as instructed:

**7 a.m. to 9 a.m.** (stomach): Just on the outside of the bottom of the knee, pat three times with your whole hand.

**9 a.m. to 11 a.m** (spleen): Rub or pat inside your knee or ankle just above the bone.

**11 a.m. to 1 p.m. and again from 1 p.m. to 3 p.m.** (heart and small intestine): Rub the top of your hand on the outside of the little finger (pinkie).

**3 p.m. to 5 p.m.** (bladder): Pinch the end of your eyebrow closest to your nose for two breaths.

**5 p.m. to 7 p.m.** (kidney): Tap the inside of your ankle four fingers width above the top of the ankle bone.

**7 p.m. to 9 p.m.** (pericardium/circulation): Rub inside middle finger (closest to index finger).

**9 p.m. to 11 p.m.** (emotional heart): Rub the top of your wrist.

**11 p.m. to 1 a.m.** (gallbladder): Rub the scalp above your ears or rub your bottom three ribs.

**1 a.m. to 3 a.m.** (liver): Rub below the right side of your chest on your ribs below your pectoralis or breast crease.

**3 a.m. to 5 a.m.** (lungs): Rub the middle of your chest at least your fingers width below your collarbone.

**5 a.m. to 7 a.m.** (large intestine): Rub the top end of the crease between your thumb and hand.

# BOOK SHANNON TO SPEAK

Shannon Eggleston is a keynote speaker and instructor known for entertaining audiences through her humor and high energy. She has a passion to impact the lives of others through speaking to serve a greater number of people throughout the world. She believes education is empowerment.

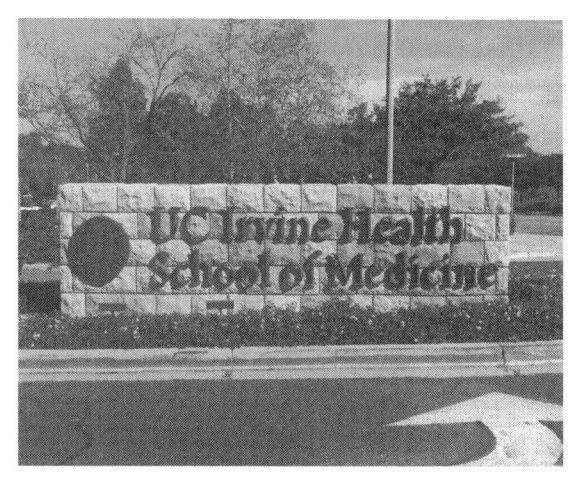

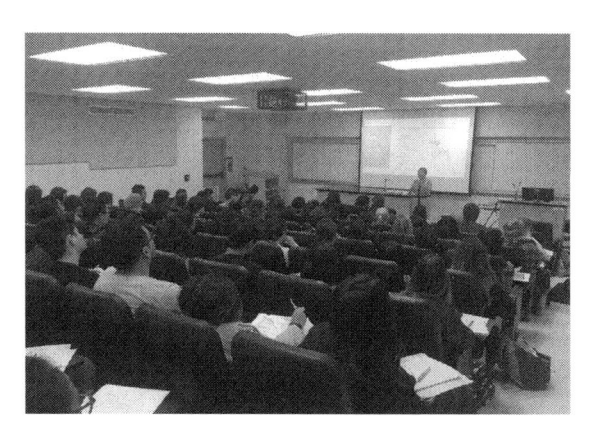

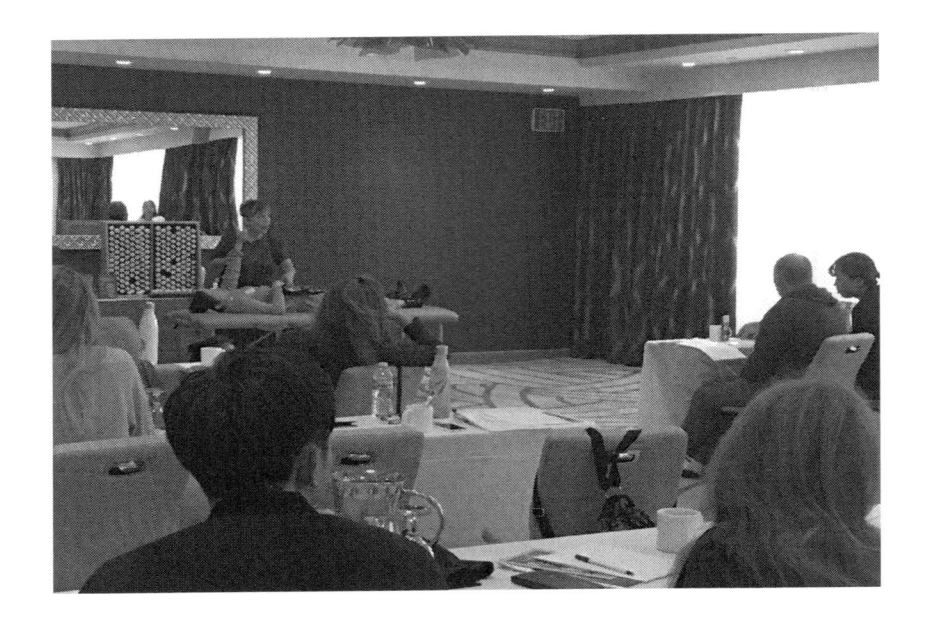

Shannon's main objective is to share how preventative health care can impact your health and well-being for a lifetime. Shannon has been speaking to a wide range of audiences: high school sport teams, nursing and pre med students at the college level, associations, women networking groups, corporations and events. She also instructs other practitioners in Nutrition Response Testing®.

To book Shannon for your next event, visit
NaturalHealingCenter.US/speaking

OR

Call 877-953-3869

# CONNECT WITH SHANNON

Website: NaturalHealingCenter.us

Email: Info@NatualHealingCenter.us

LinkedIn: LinkedIn.com/in/shannon-eggleston-701612a/

Facebook: Facebook.com/NaturalHealingCenterandInstitute

Instagram: Instagram.com/NaturalHealingOC

Youtube: https://bit.ly/2EKtGJM

# I'D LOVE TO HEAR FROM YOU

**amazon**

★★★★★

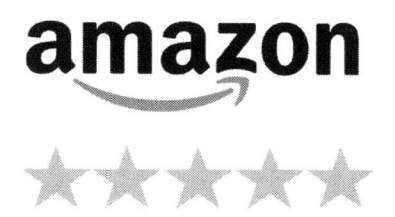

Thanks to everyone who bought this book.

Many of you are our clients already and have experienced great success.

For those of you who haven't been to the office yet, to increase your health and healing, what do you think of the book?

I'd love to hear from you!

To leave a review visit: https://amzn.to/2qxZ6hk

Made in the USA
Columbia, SC
22 April 2019